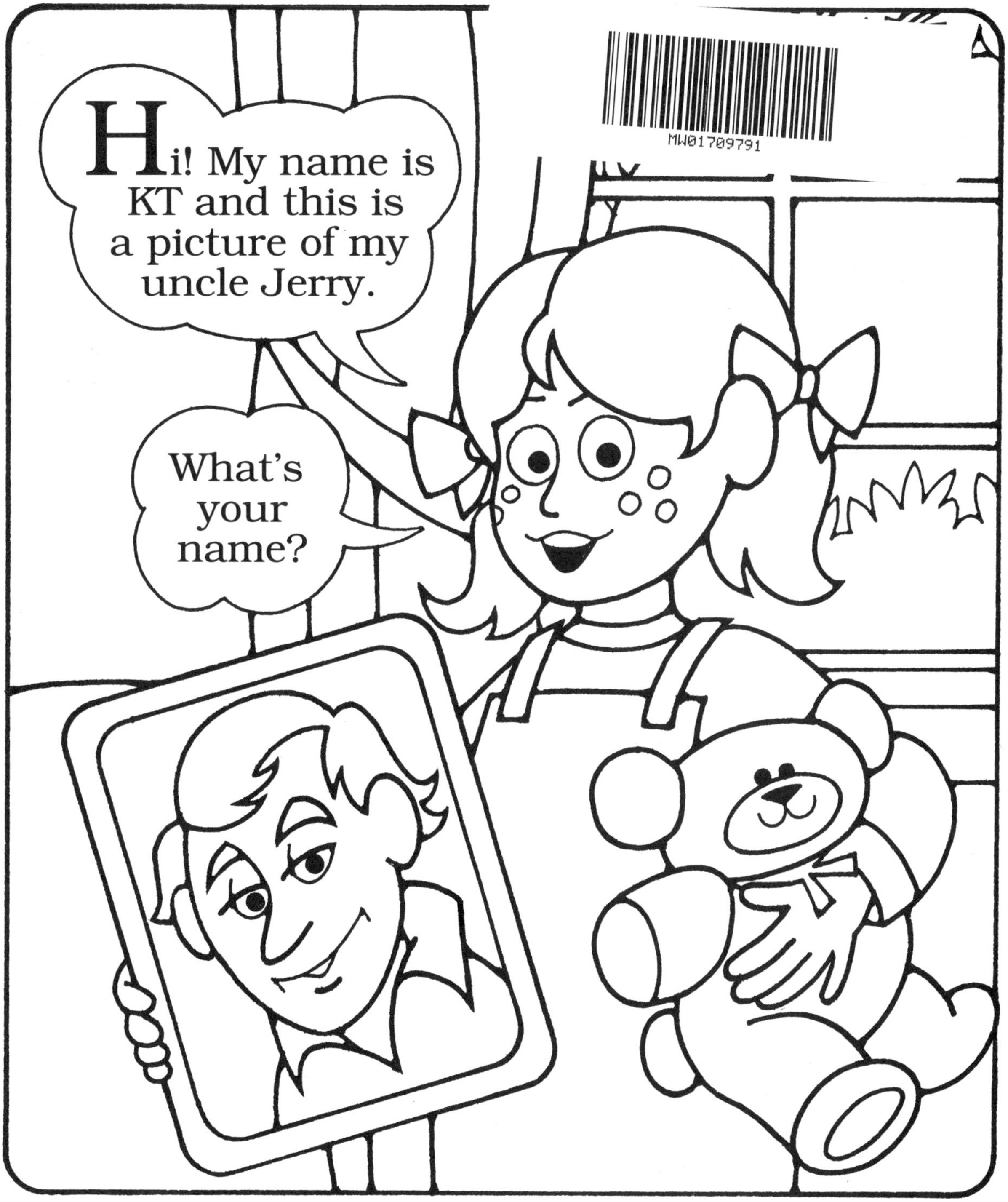
Hi! My name is KT and this is a picture of my uncle Jerry.
What's your name?

Your name

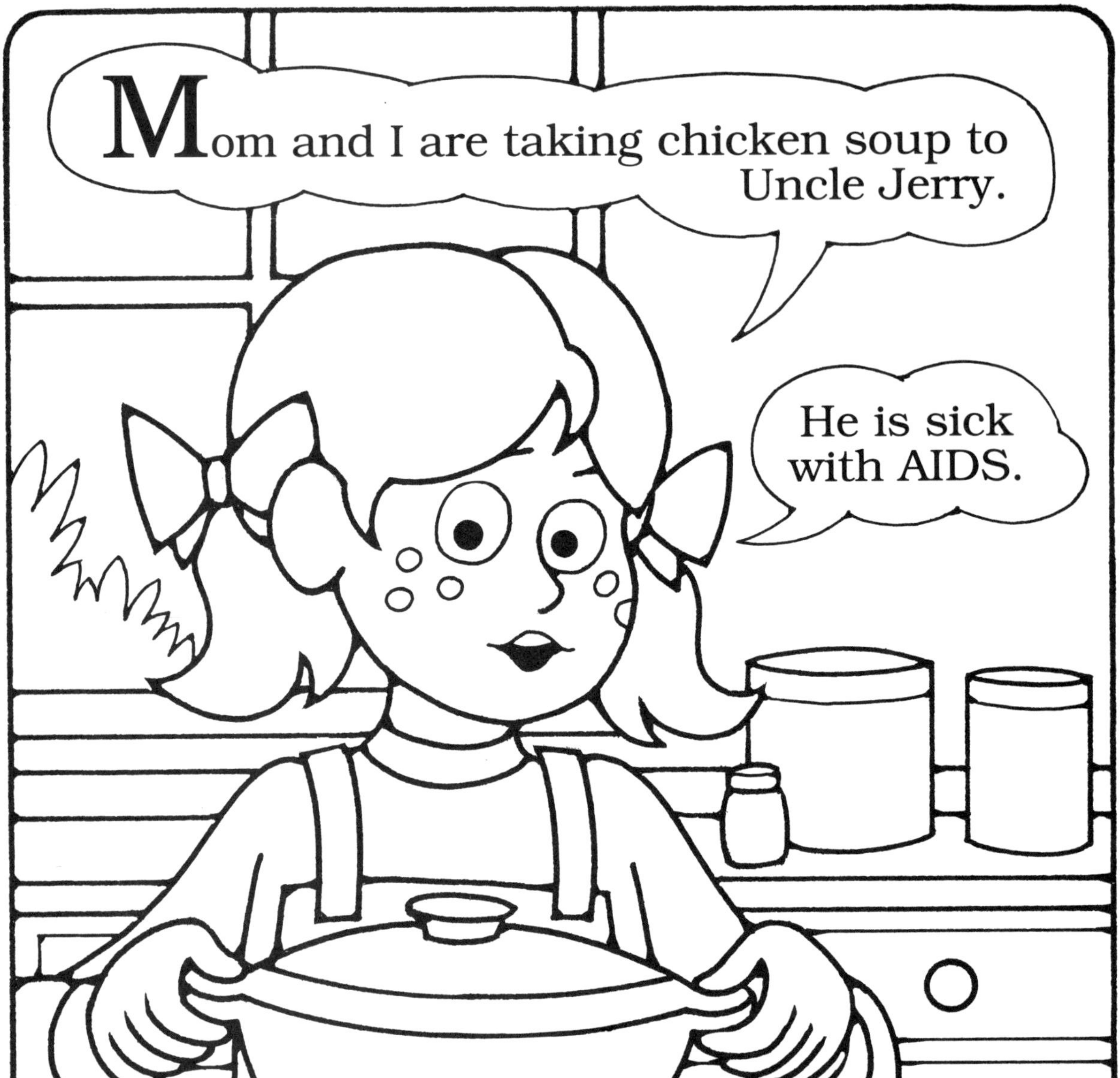

*What have you heard about AIDS?*______

______

______

Please draw a face showing how you feel about AIDS.

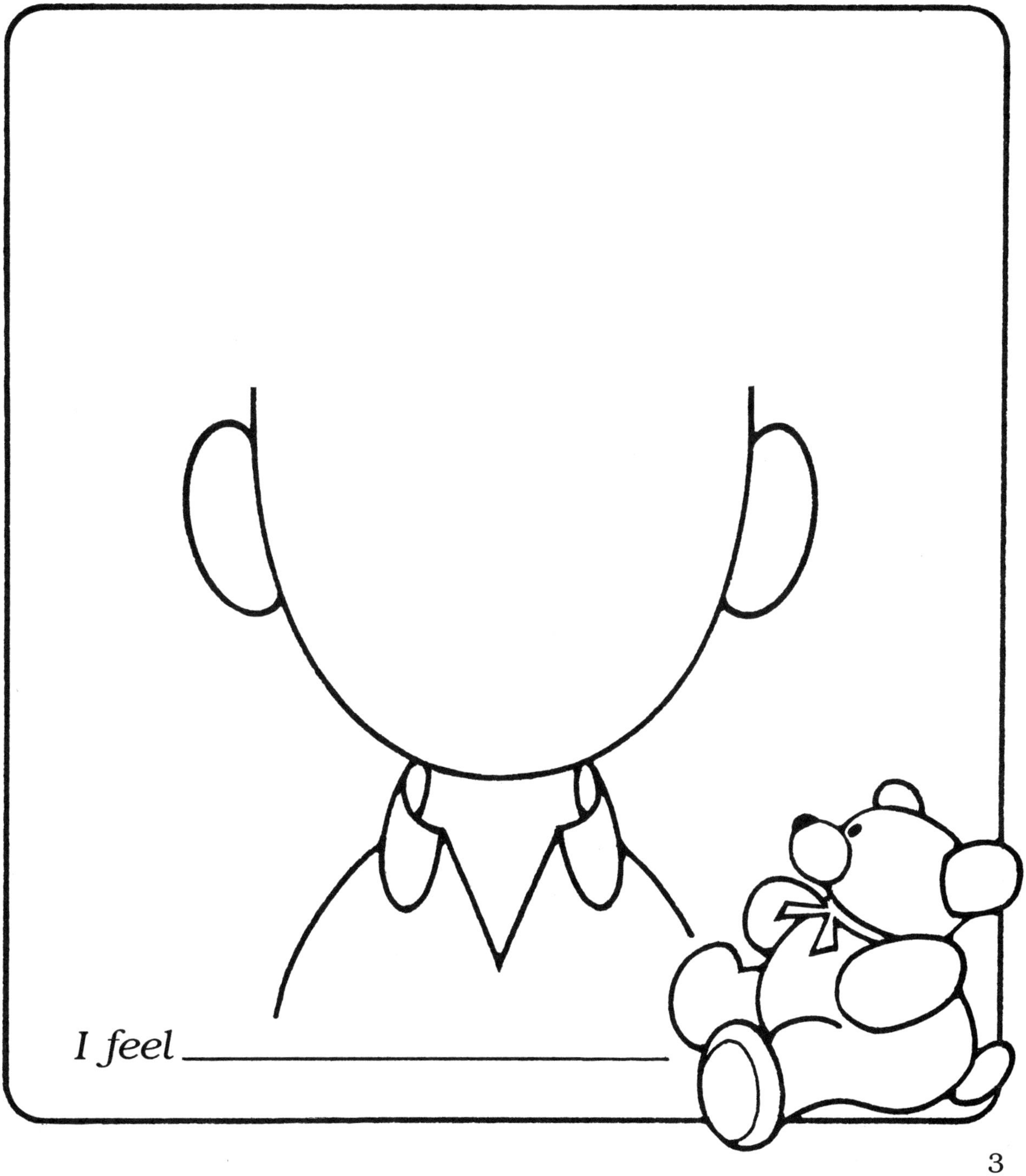

I feel ______________________________

AIDS is a disease caused by a tiny life form called a virus. It is too small for the eye to see.

The name of this virus is HIV.
It is also called "the AIDS virus."

The virus lives in Uncle Jerry's body.
It makes it very hard for him to stay healthy.

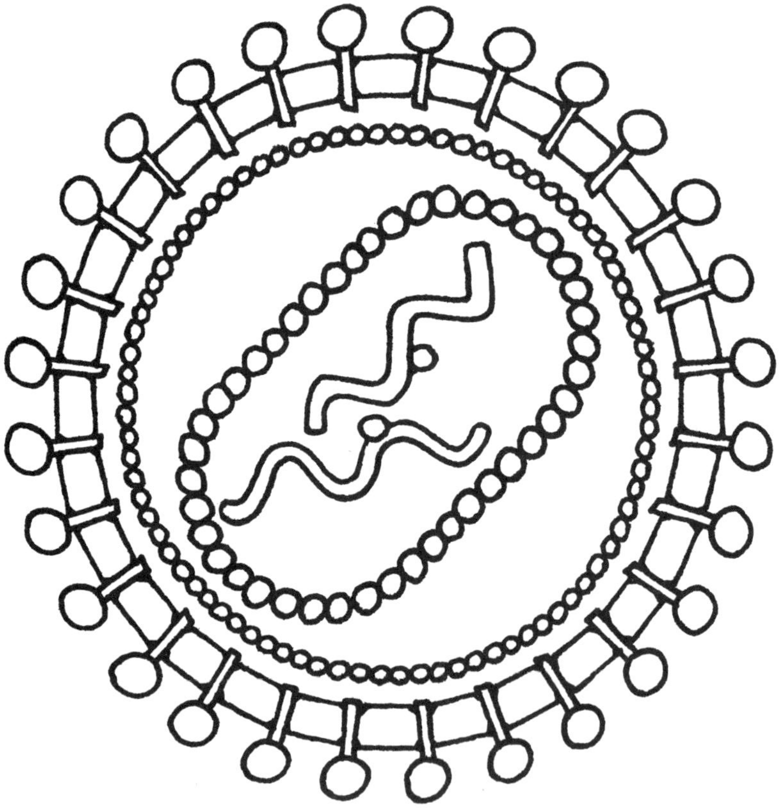

This is what the AIDS virus looks like.
You can color it if you want to.

When you and I get sick, our bodies usually heal quickly.

When Uncle Jerry gets sick, it is hard for his body to heal itself.

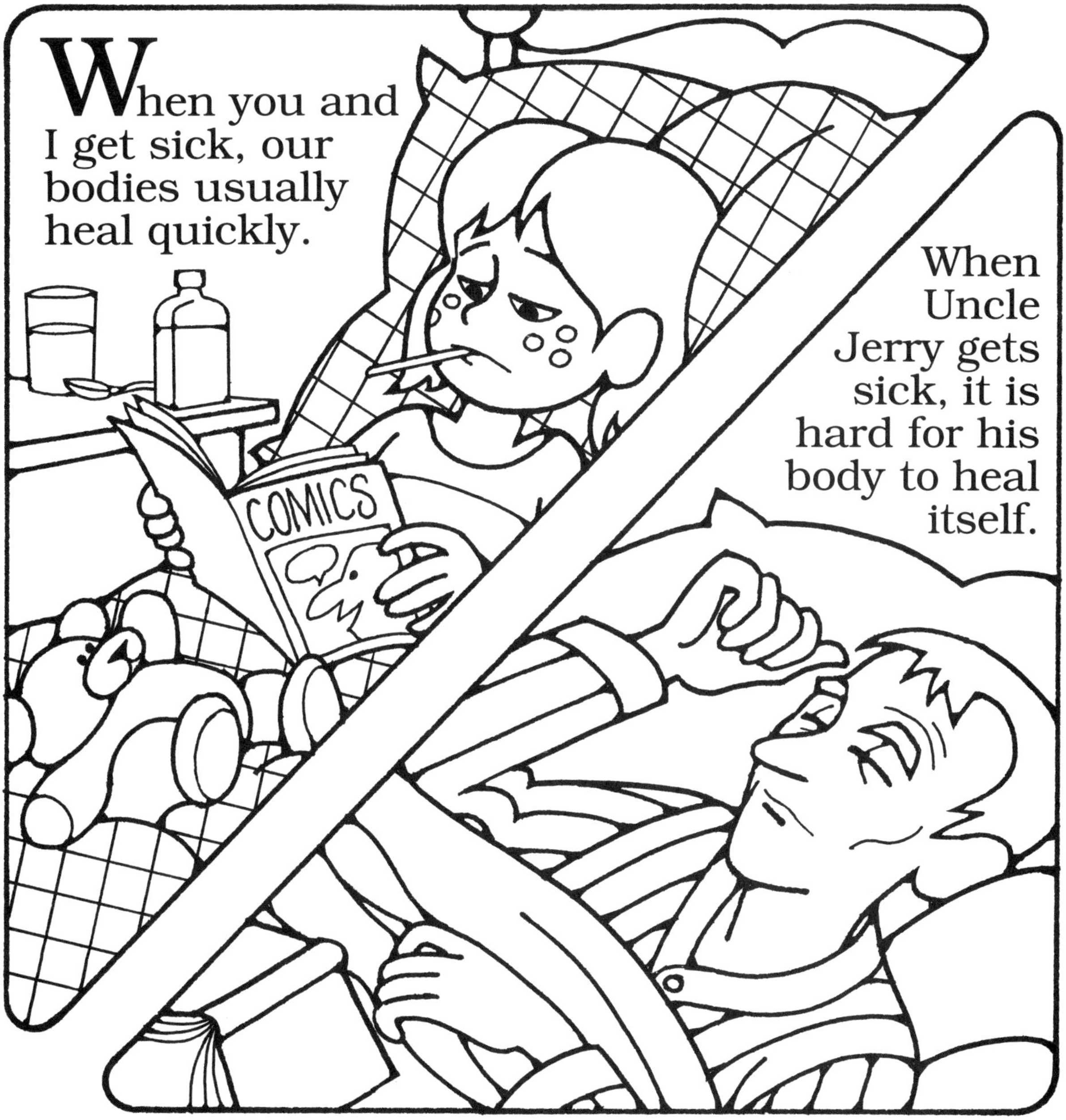

Remember a time when you were sick.
What did it feel like? ____________________

____

____

Mom and I don't want to give any new germs to Uncle Jerry.

We waited until our colds were gone before visiting him.

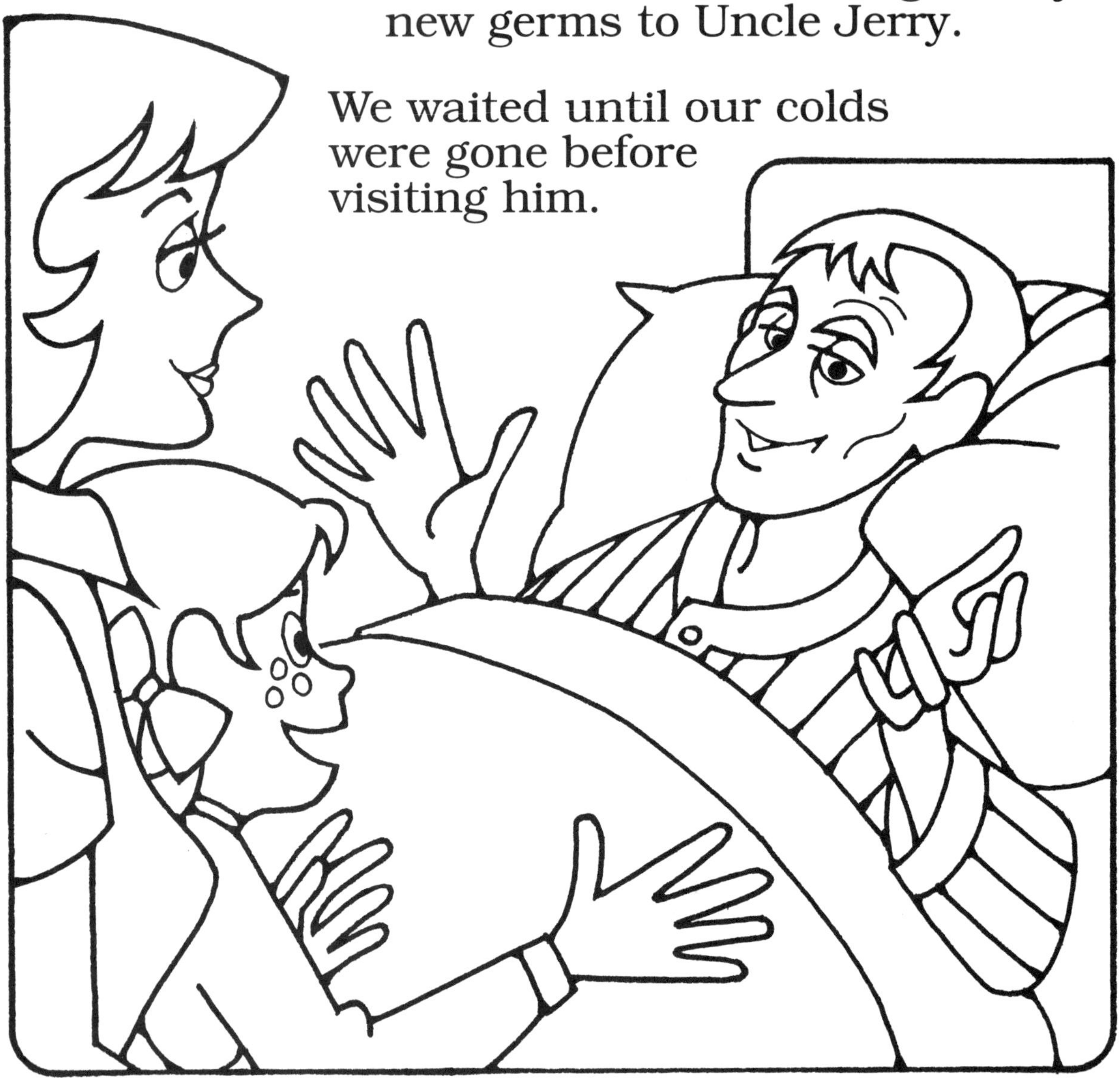

Name two ways to avoid giving germs to other people.

1) ____________________________________

2) ____________________________________

I wash my hands with soap and warm water so I will not give Uncle Jerry any germs when I touch him.

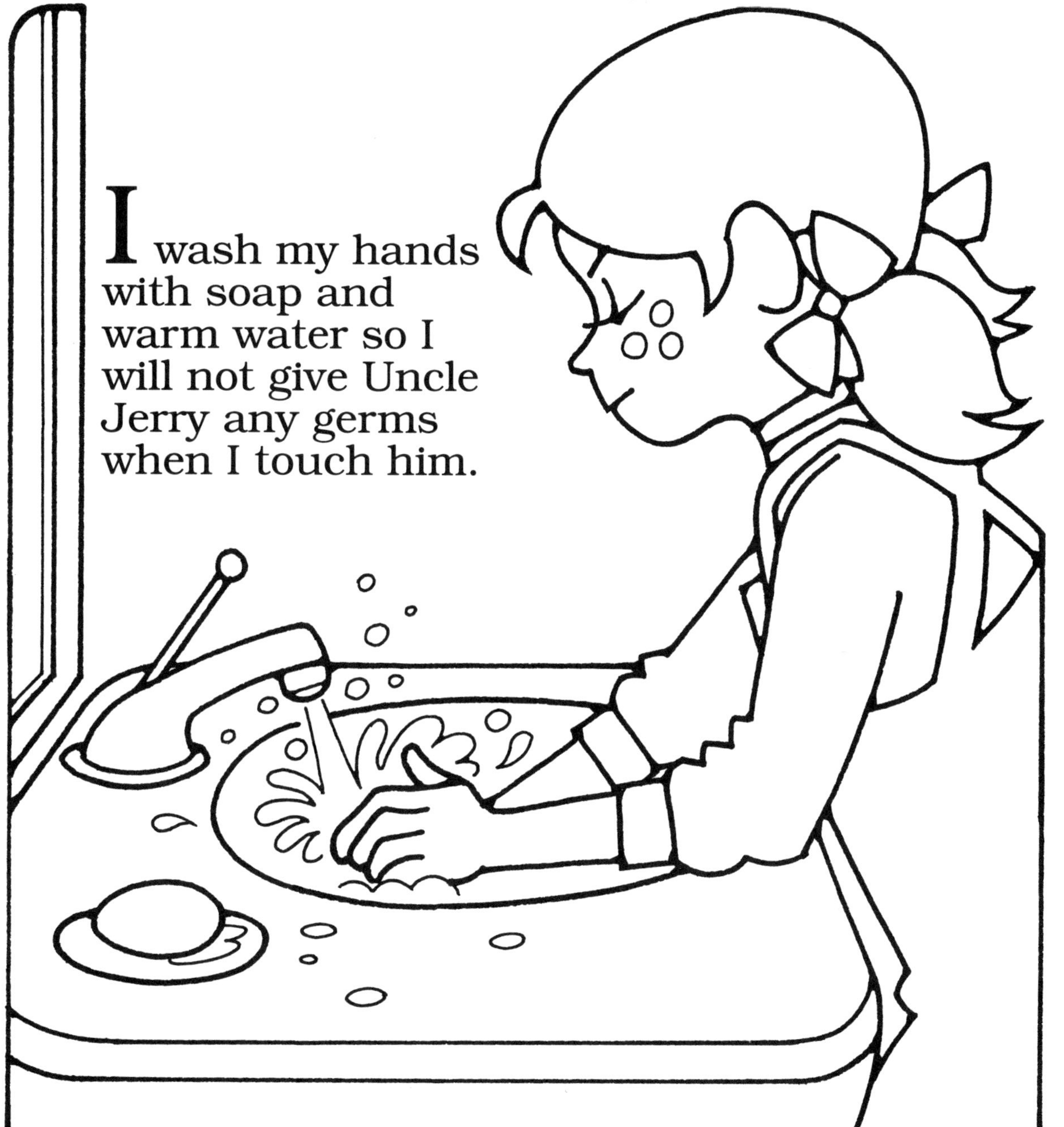

At what times do you wash your hands?

____

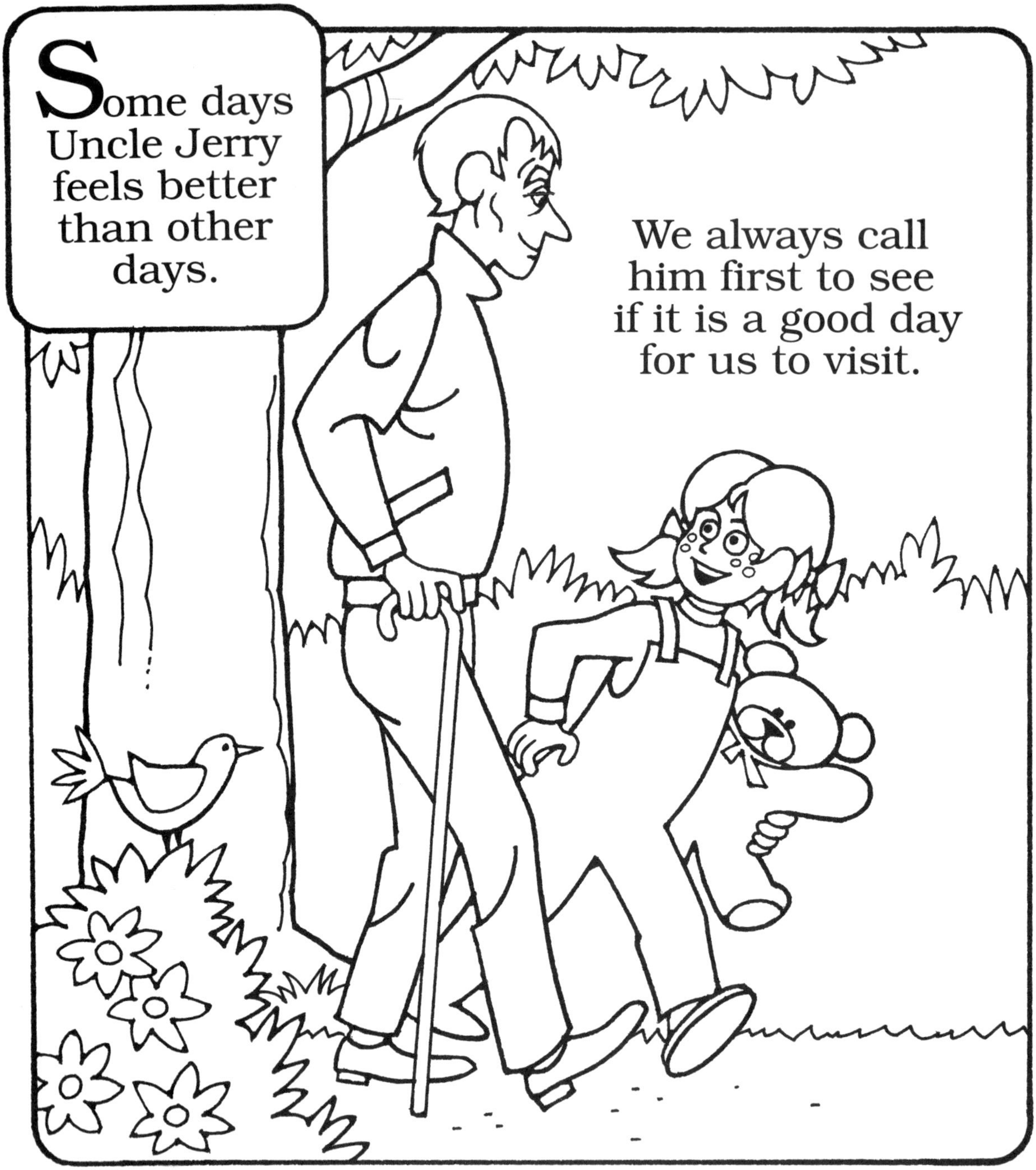

*How would you feel about visiting someone who has AIDS?*________________________

____

I like to visit Uncle Jerry.

We drink milk
and eat chocolate
chip cookies.

Sometimes we
even have ice cream.

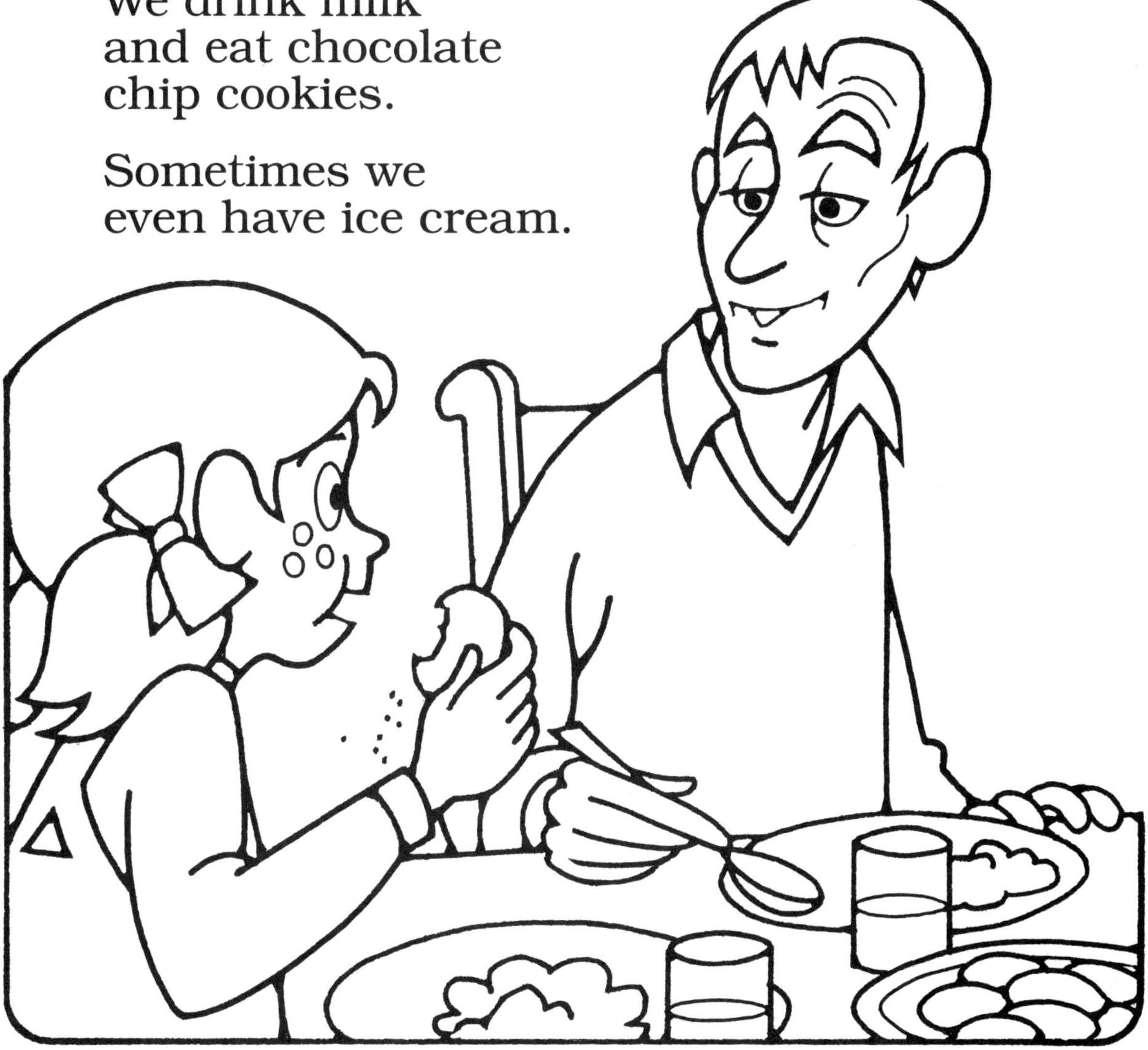

*How would you feel about sitting next to someone who has AIDS?*____________

____

____

When Uncle Jerry is feeling bad,
I hold his hand and tell him jokes.

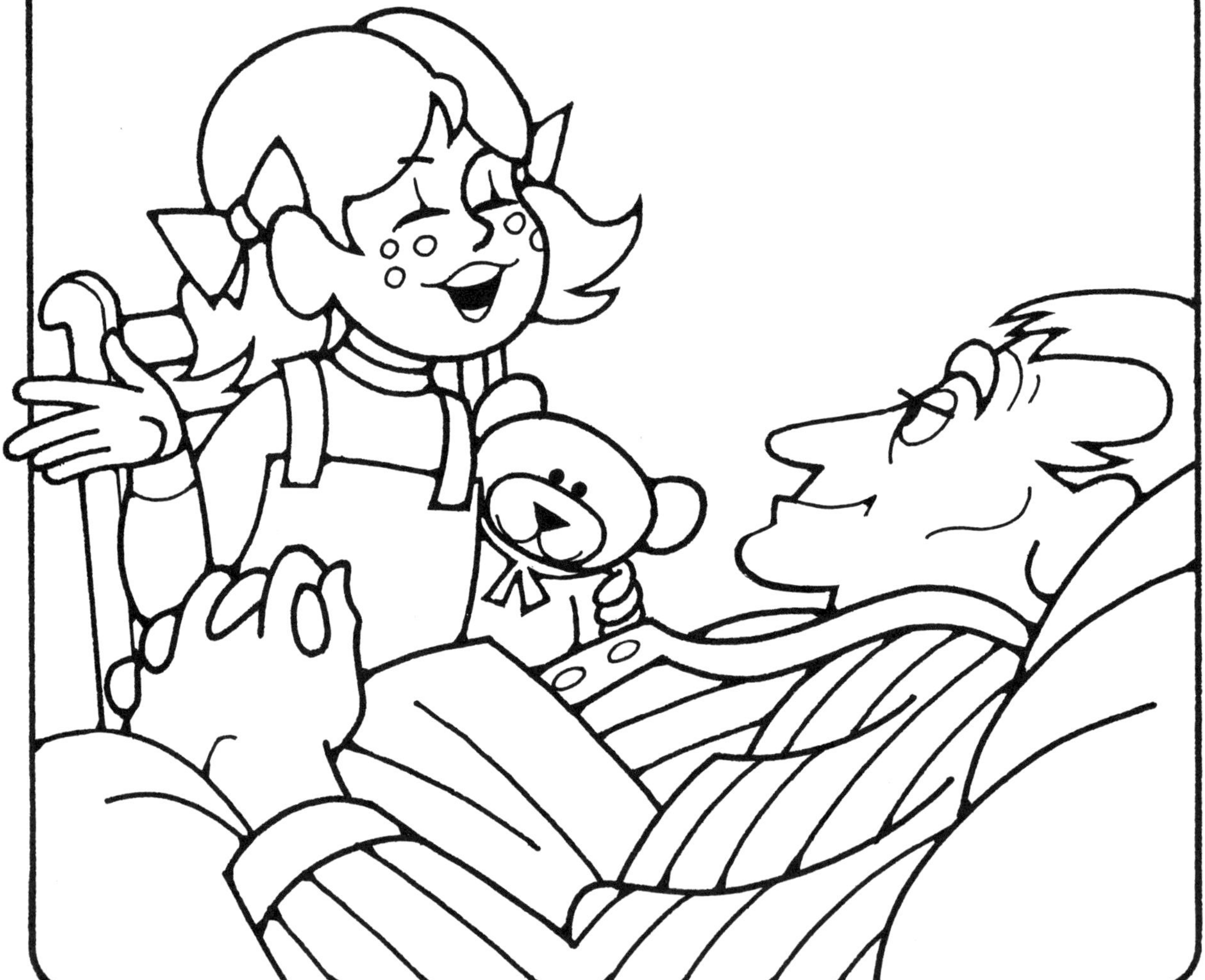

What animal can jump higher than a house?

All animals — because houses can't jump.

I don't have to worry about getting AIDS from hugging Uncle Jerry.

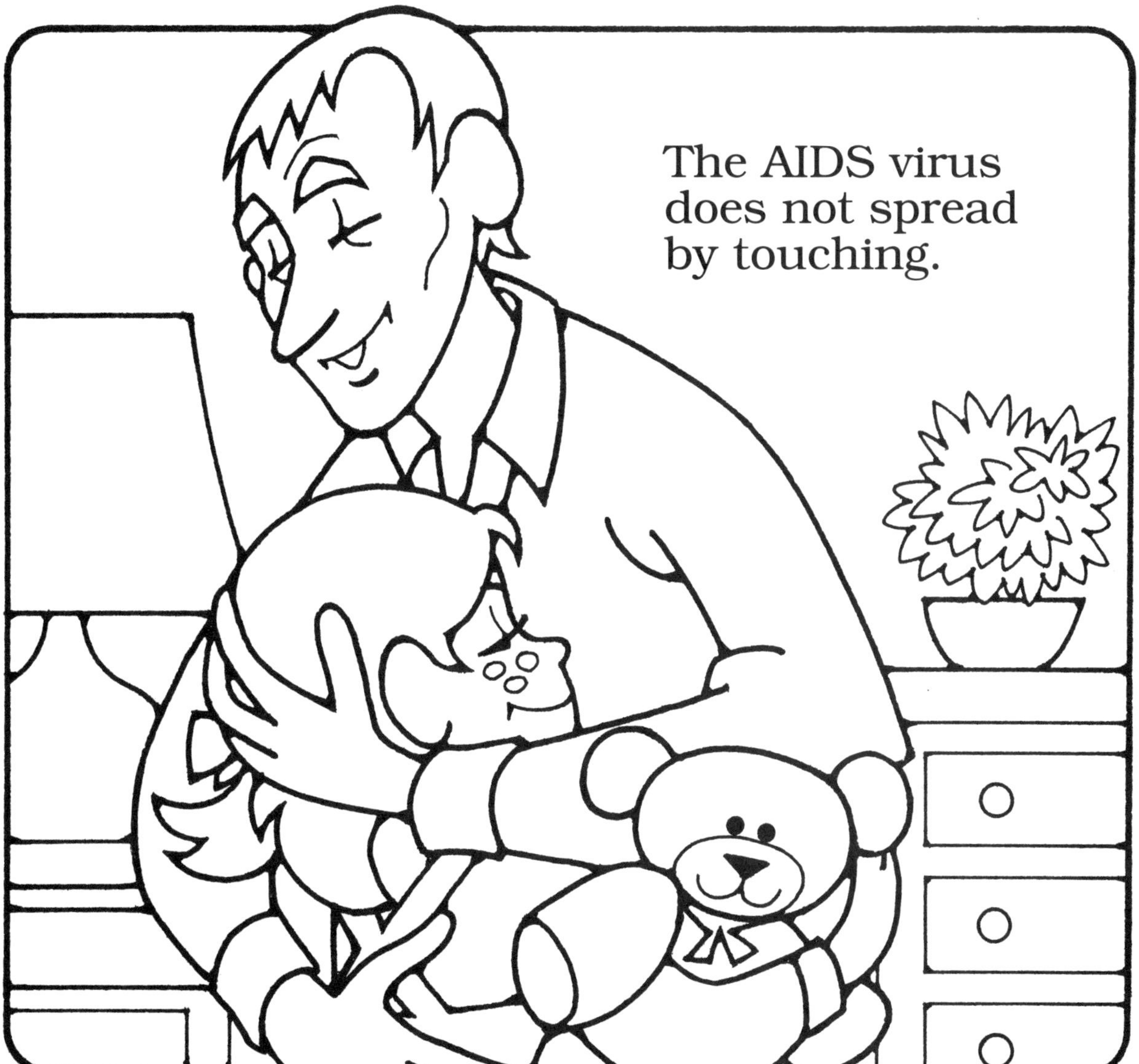

*How would you feel about touching someone who has AIDS?*____________________________

____

AIDS is hard to catch.

The AIDS virus does not travel through
the air like the cold germ does.
It dies when exposed to air.

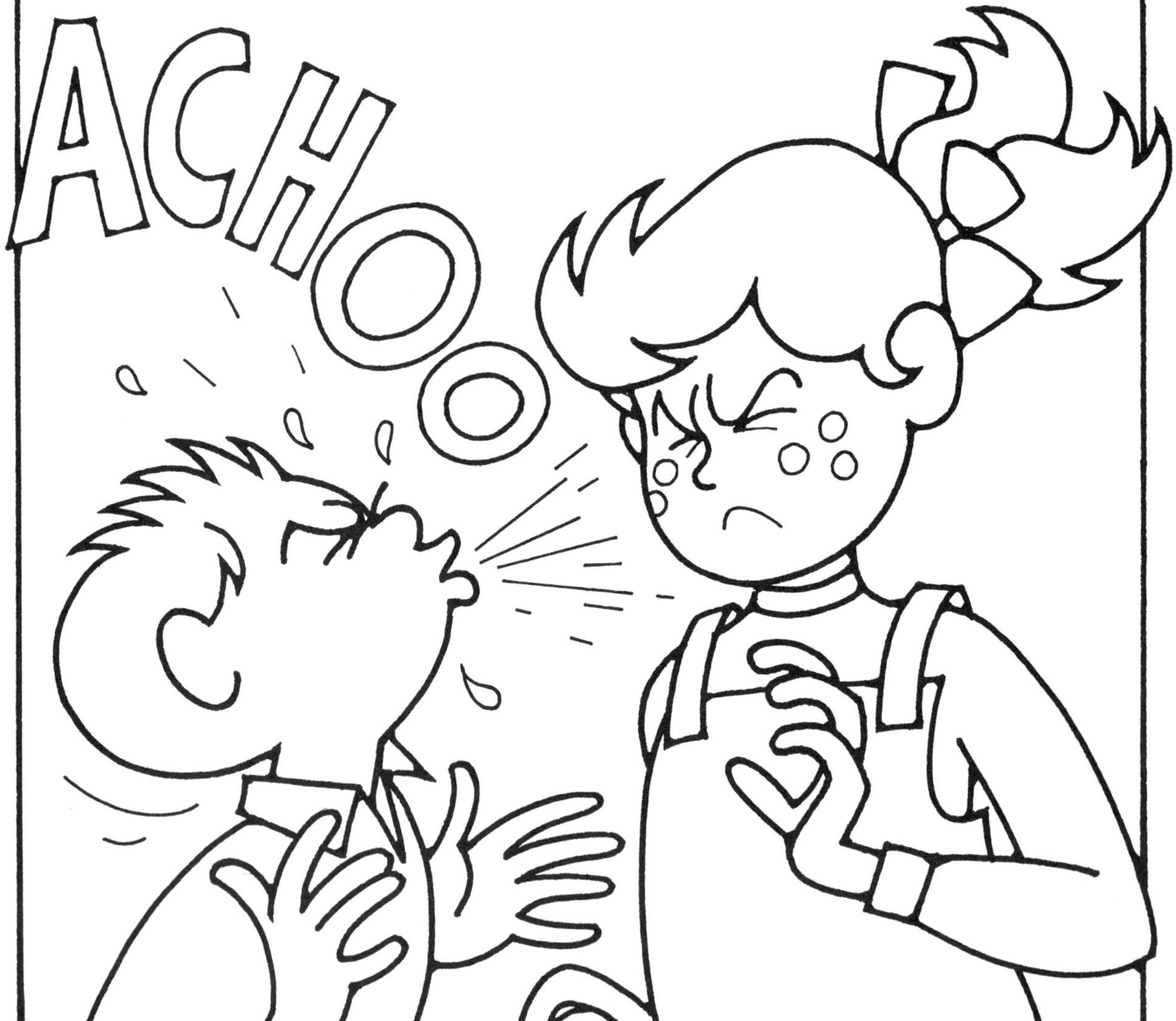

The AIDS virus lives in blood and other body fluids. There is no danger of catching AIDS from spit or sweat or tears.

It is safe to play with a person who has AIDS.

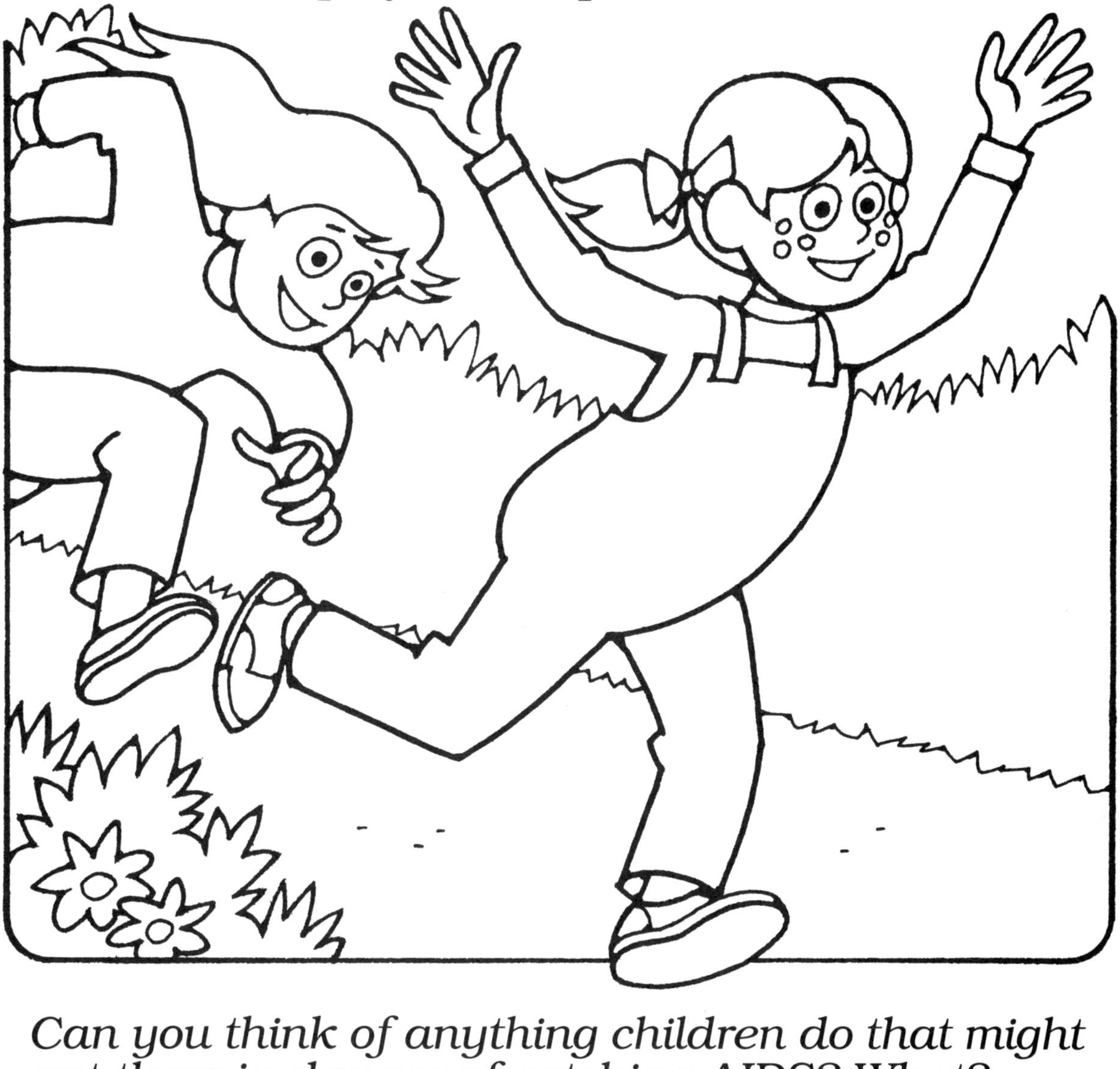

Can you think of anything children do that might put them in danger of catching AIDS? What?

Mom and I always help clean the house when we visit Uncle Jerry.

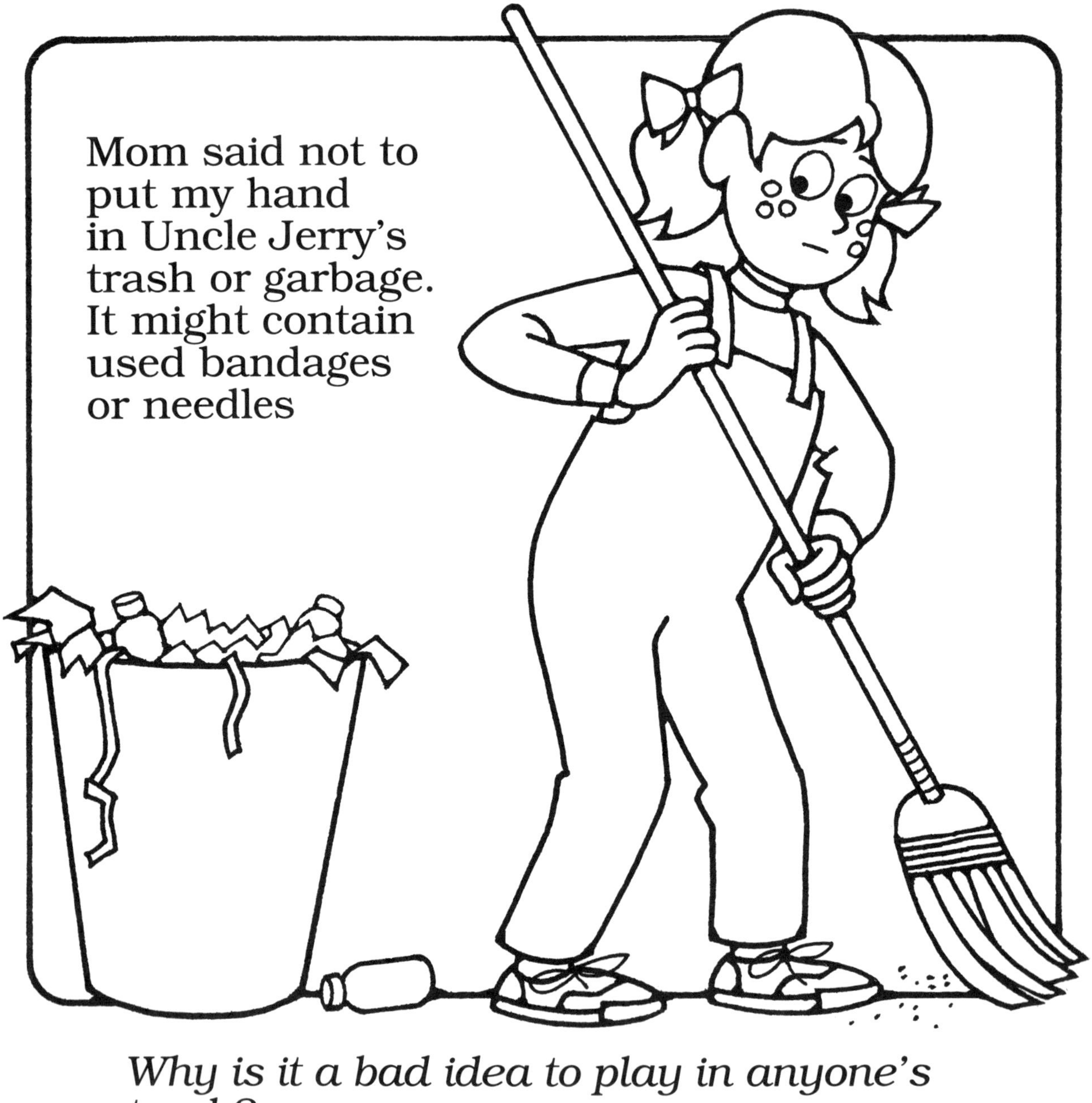

Why is it a bad idea to play in anyone's trash? ______________________________

____

Doctors give Uncle Jerry lots of pills and shots. The medicine helps his body fight AIDS, but it doesn't cure him.

Mom told me never to touch the medicine.

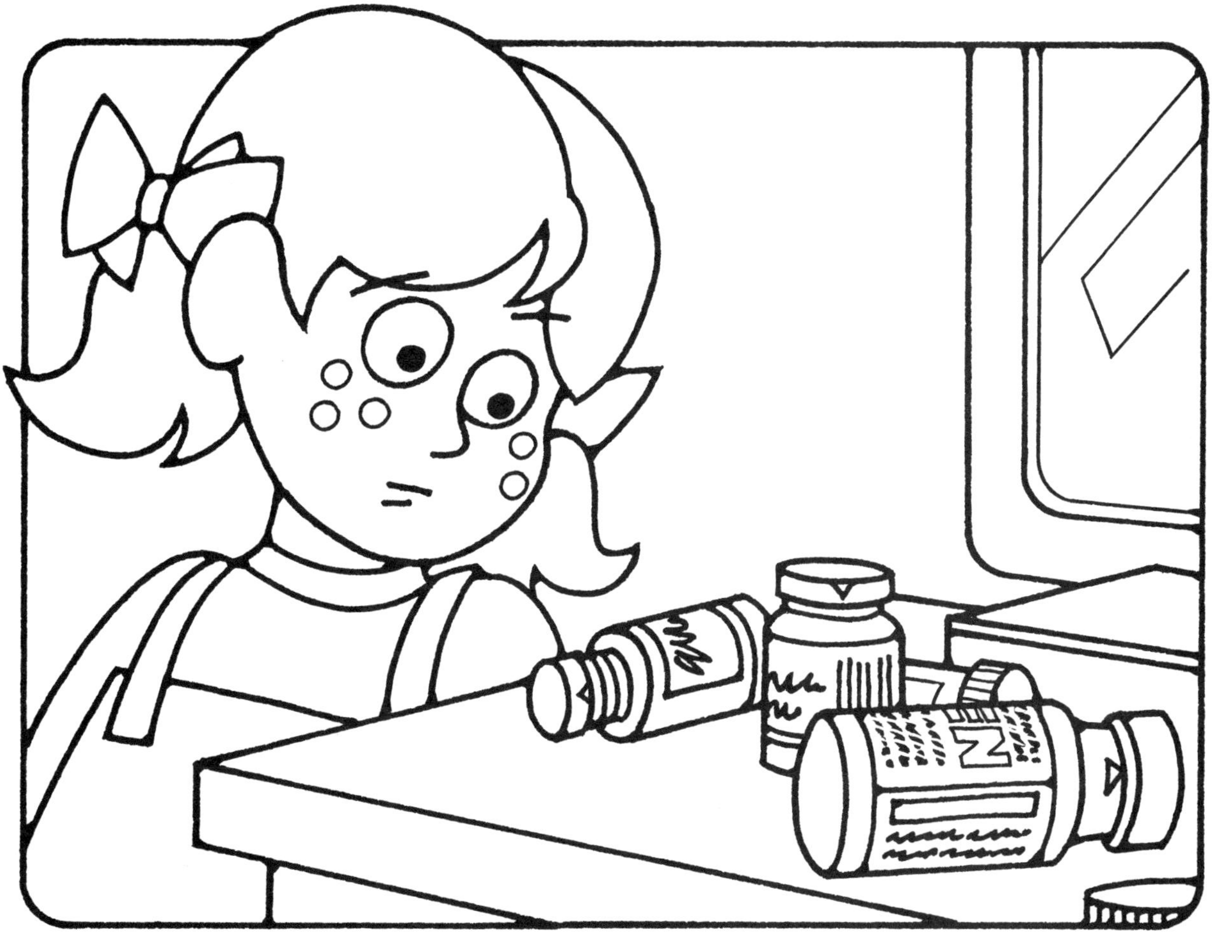

*Why do you think KT's mom said not to touch the medicine?*____________________

____

____

Even though Uncle Jerry takes medicine, he still gets sick.

One of these days he may die unless a cure for AIDS is found soon.

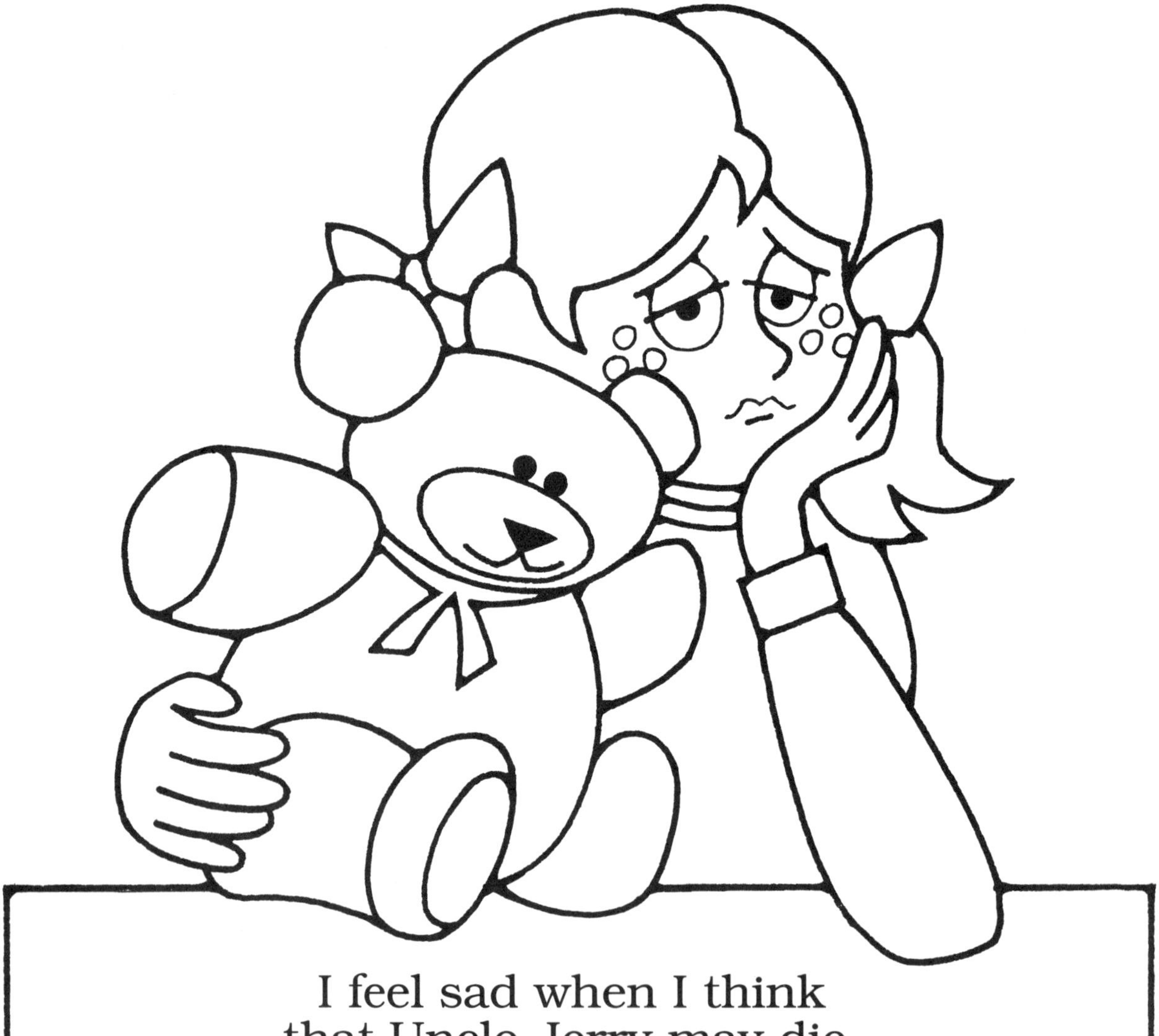

I feel sad when I think that Uncle Jerry may die.

Many years ago, terrible diseases killed lots of people. Scientists today know how to cure many of those diseases.

Several medicines have already been found that will help Uncle Jerry stay healthy longer.

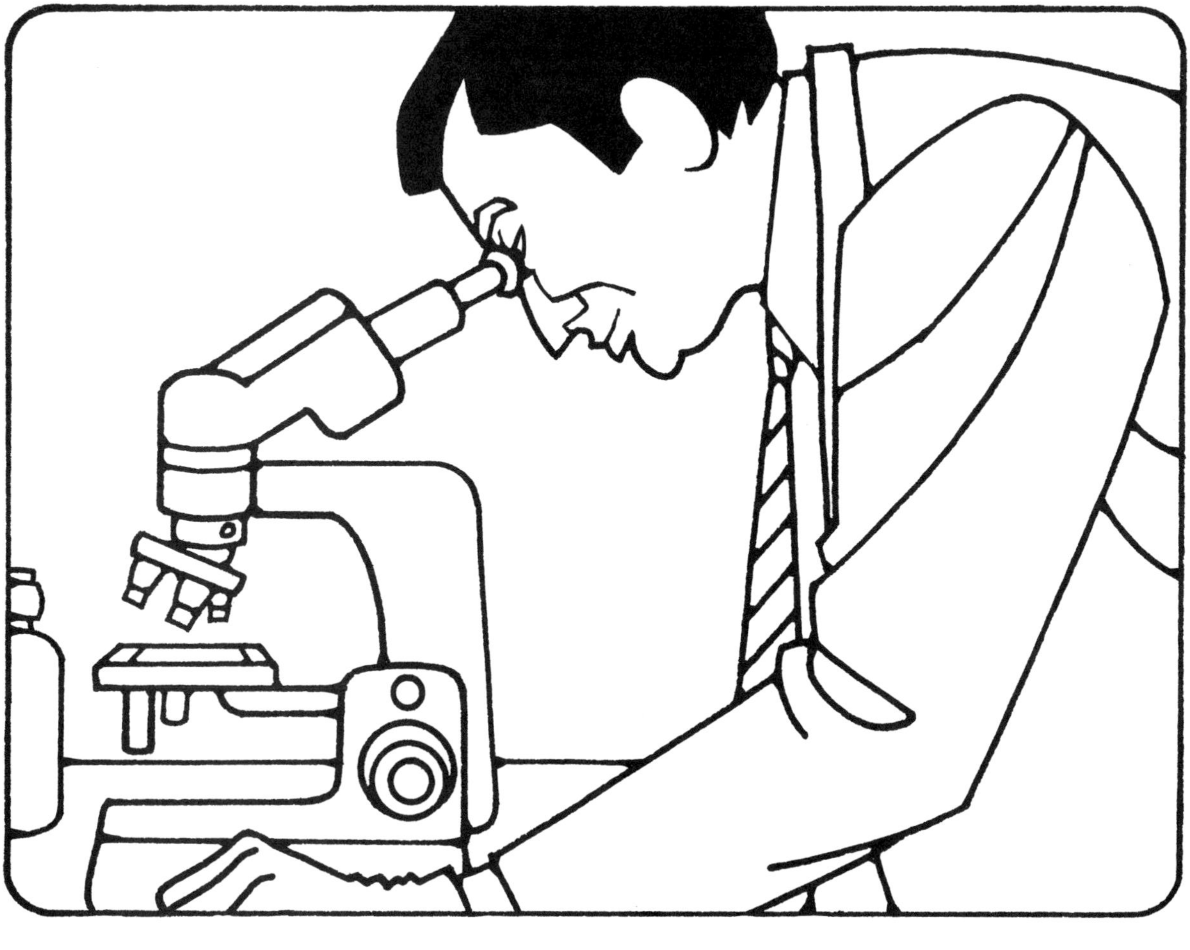

Name a disease for which scientists have discovered a prevention or cure. ________

____

Uncle Jerry is not the only person I know with AIDS. One of my teachers also has AIDS. She doesn't look sick at all.

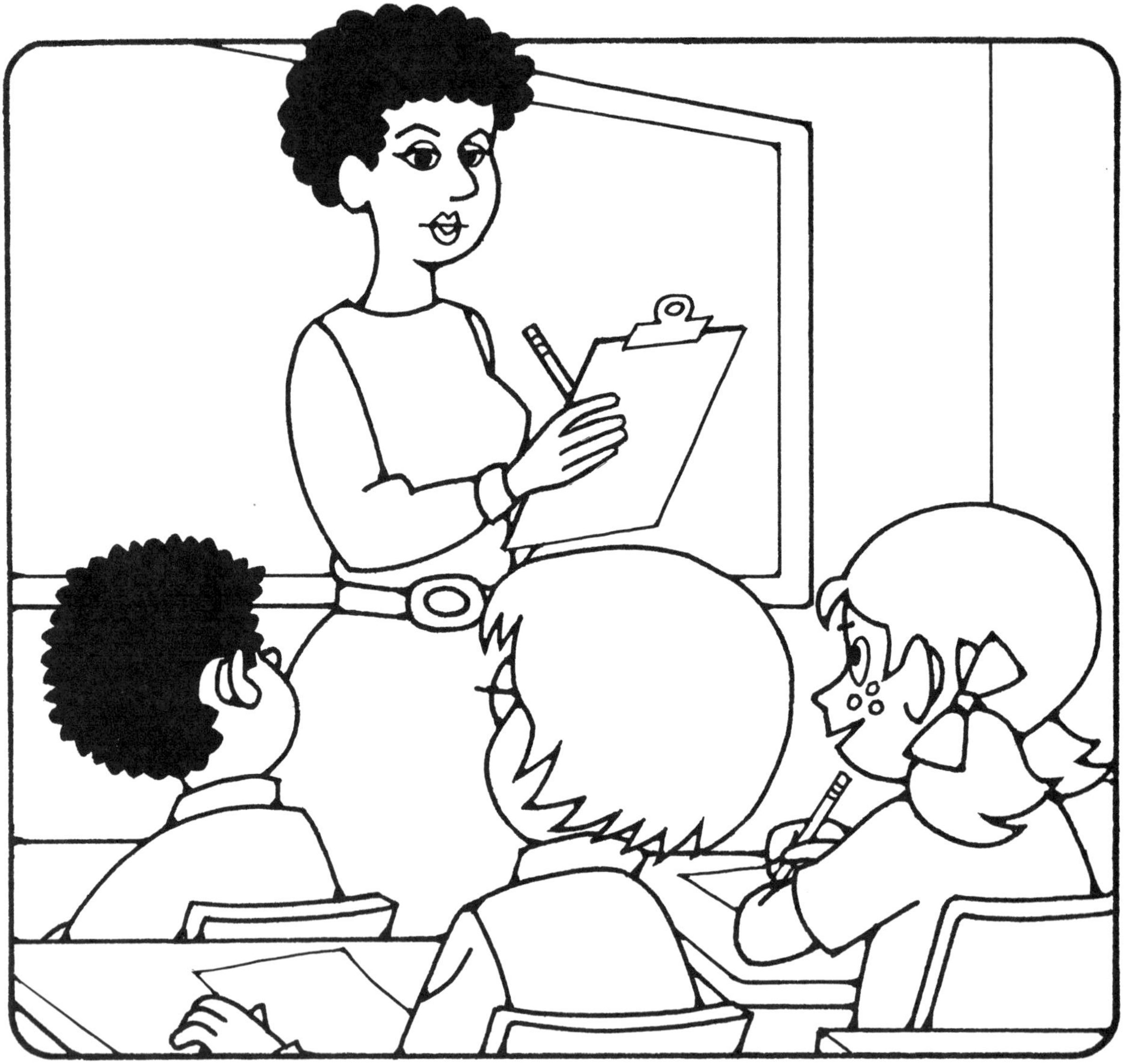

People with AIDS look like everyone else. Sometimes they don't even know they have AIDS.

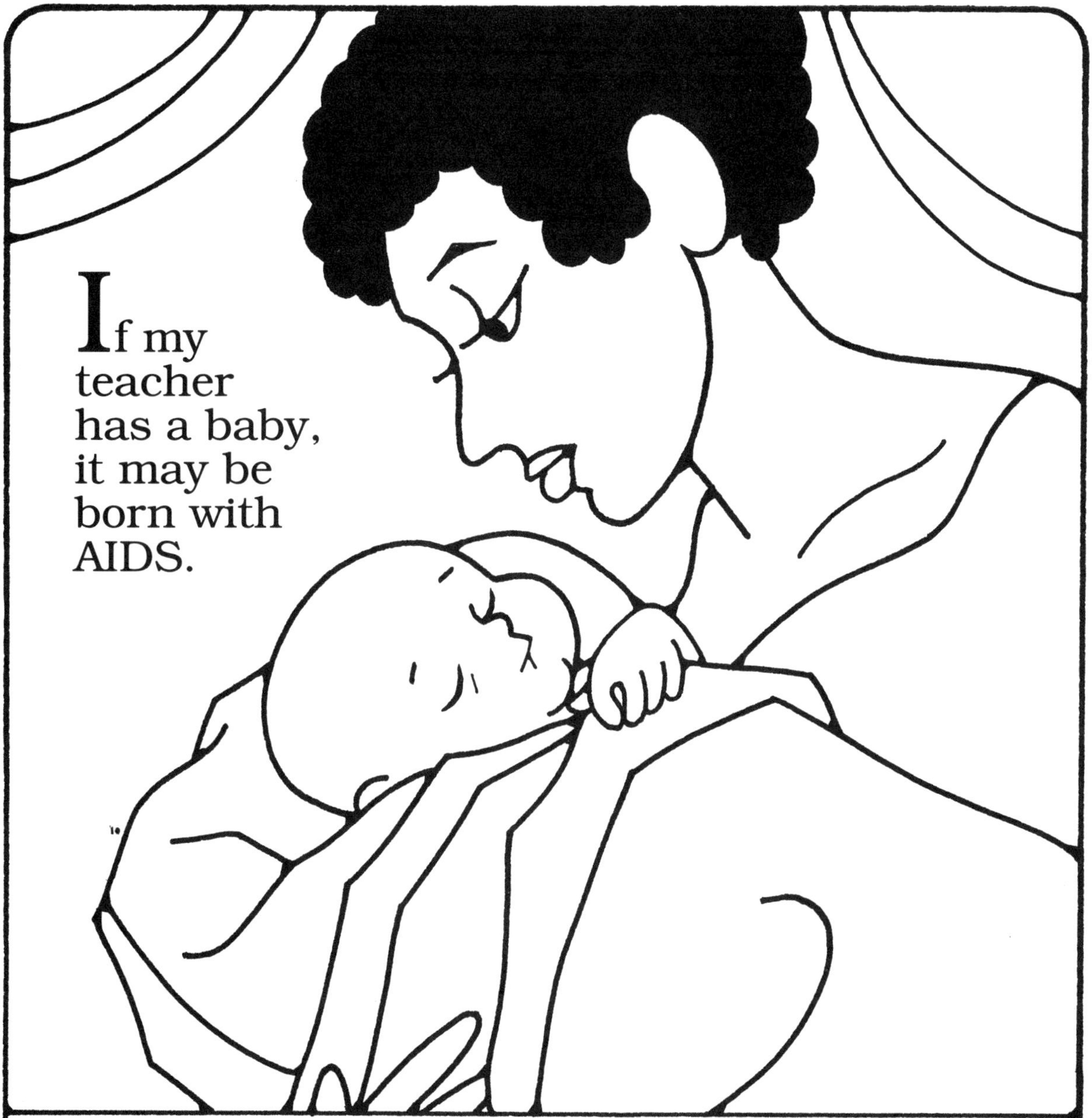

If my teacher has a baby, it may be born with AIDS.

How can a baby catch AIDS from its mother?

____

____

Some parents do not want their kids to be around my teacher with AIDS.

This is hard for me to understand. She is my favorite teacher.

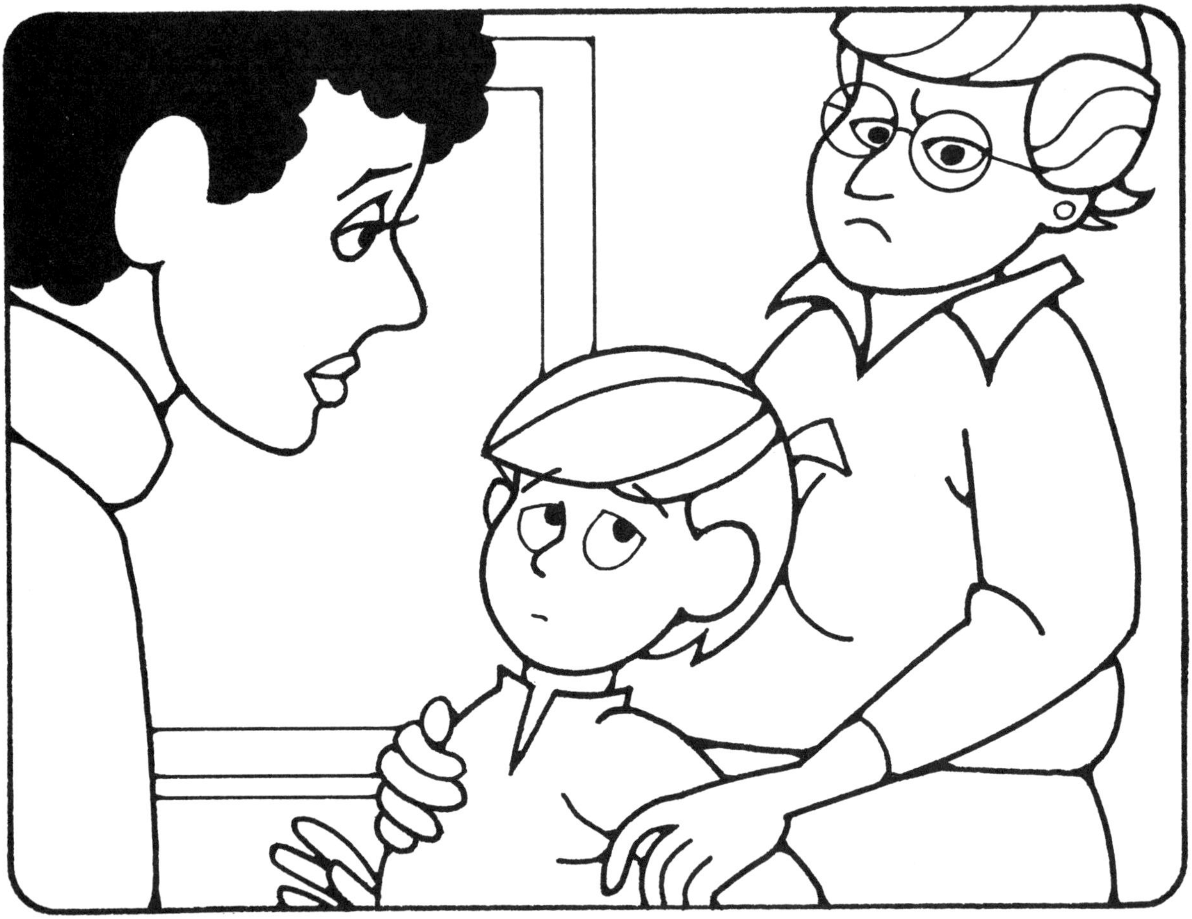

*Why are some people mean to people who have AIDS?*______________________________

____

____

All kinds of people get AIDS.

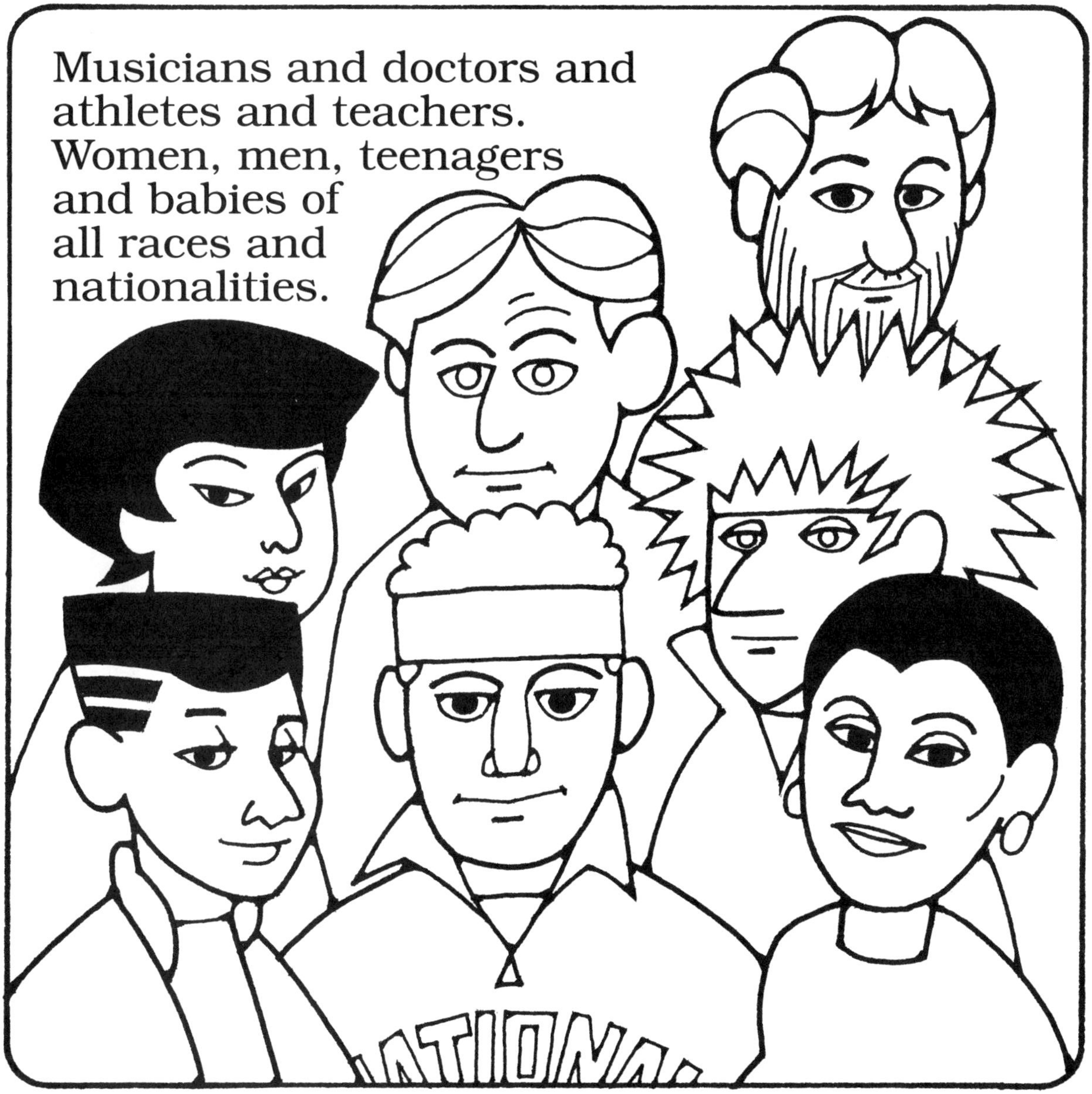

Who have you heard about who has AIDS?

____

Color those faces that show how you feel toward people who have AIDS.

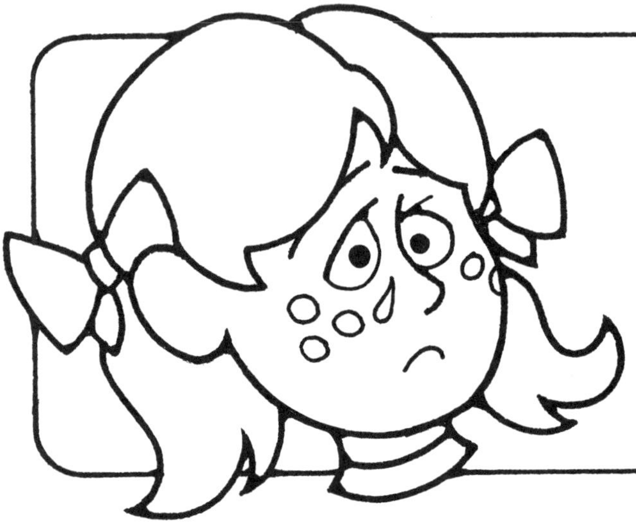

Sad that they hurt.

Afraid of getting AIDS.

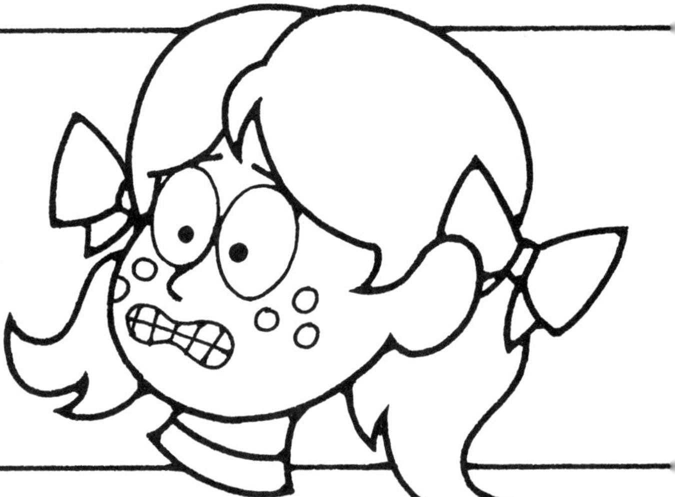

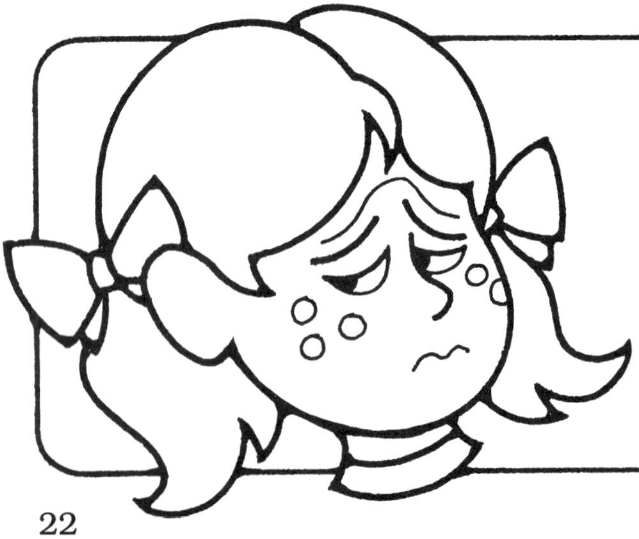

Guilty for feeling good when others are so sick.

Angry at them for having AIDS.

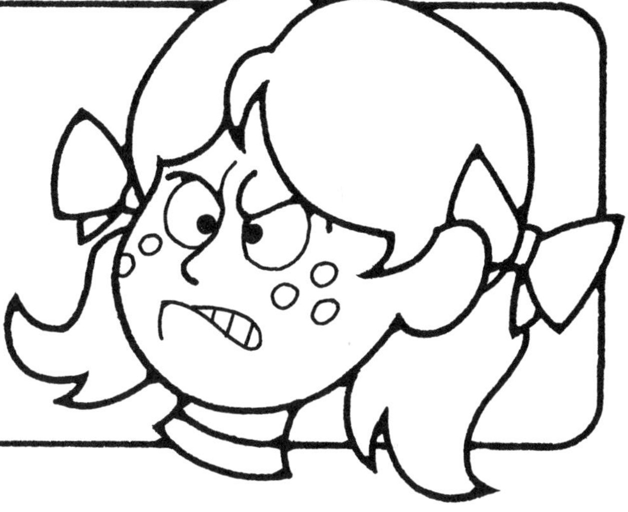

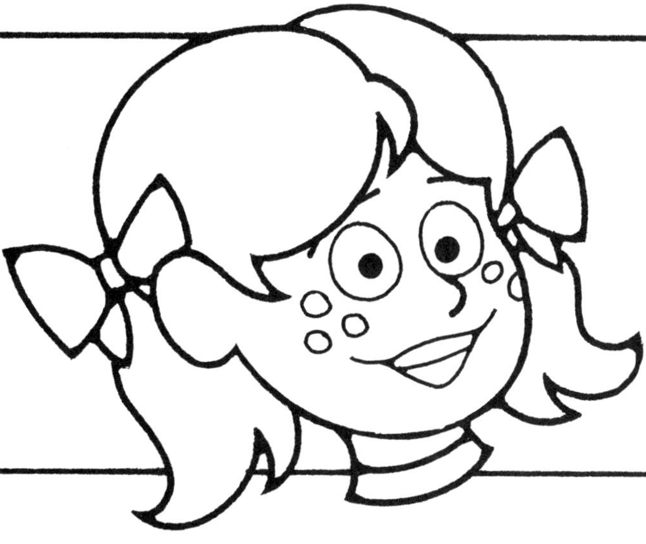

Wanting to help them.

I feel ____________________

____

____

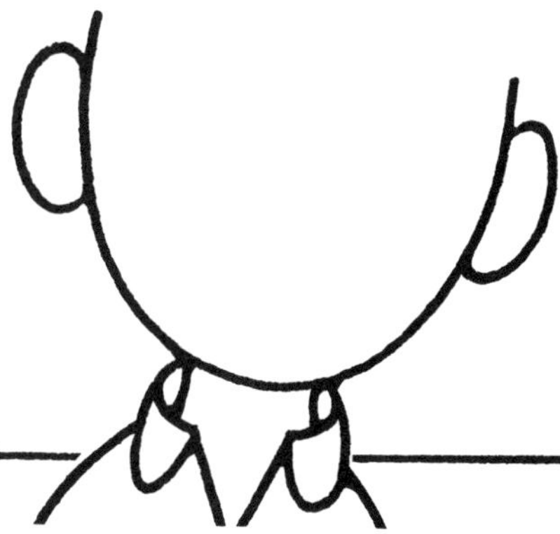

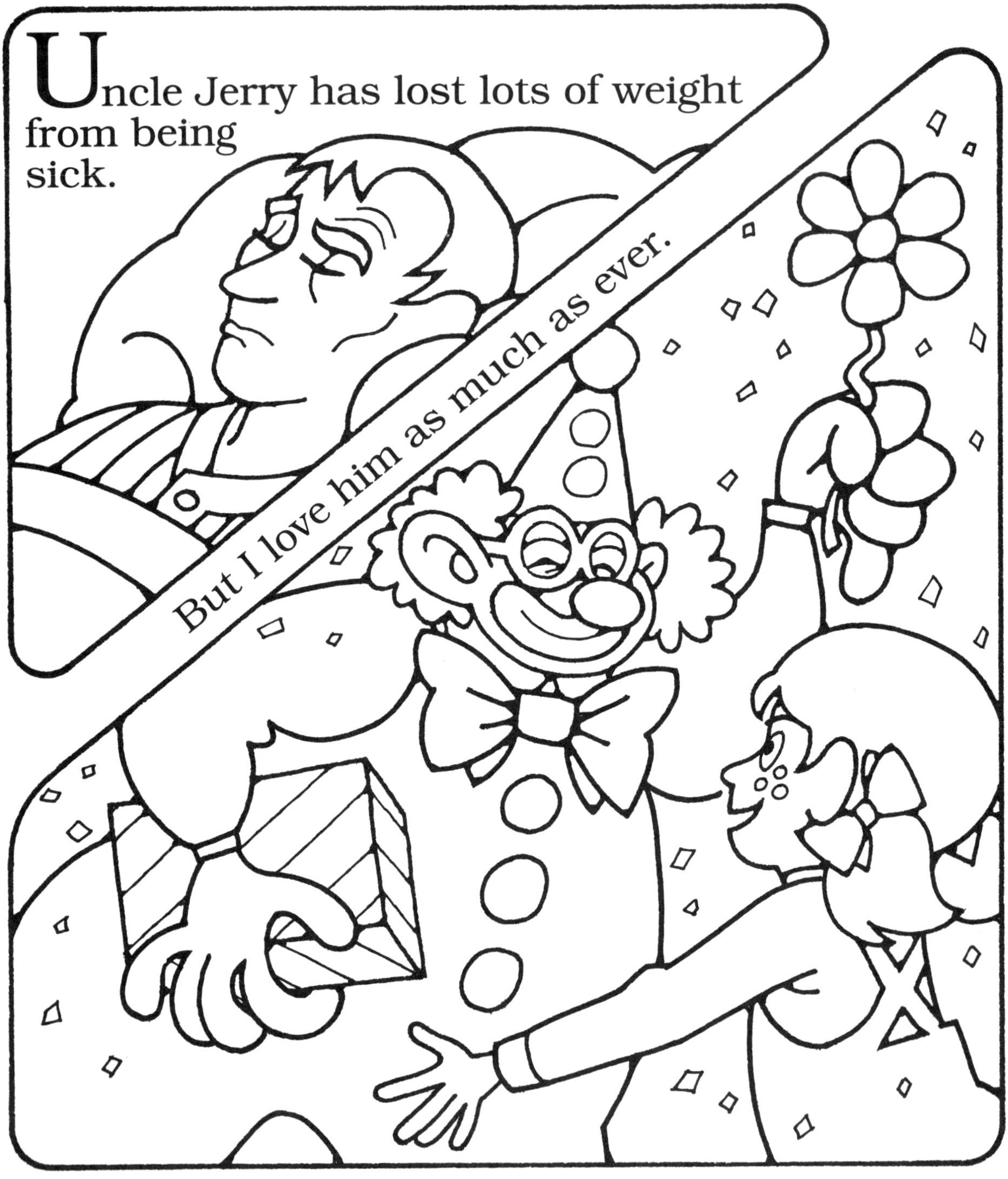

He is the same wonderful person who played a clown at my last birthday.

My family has grown much closer since Uncle Jerry became sick.

We realize how important we are to each other.

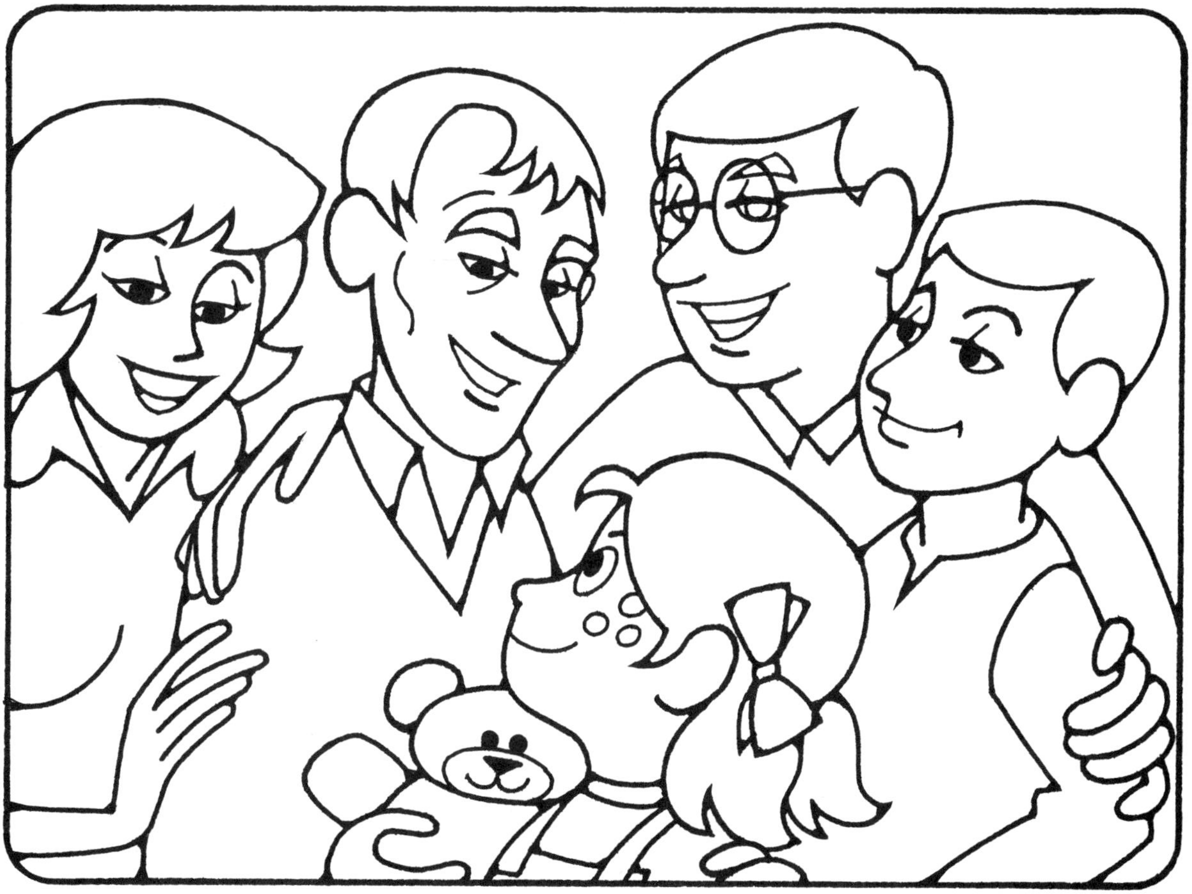

What friends and relatives do you feel close to?

____

____

____

I am thankful for each day that Uncle Jerry is alive.

Sometimes I call him on the telephone just to hear his voice.

Each visit with him is very special.

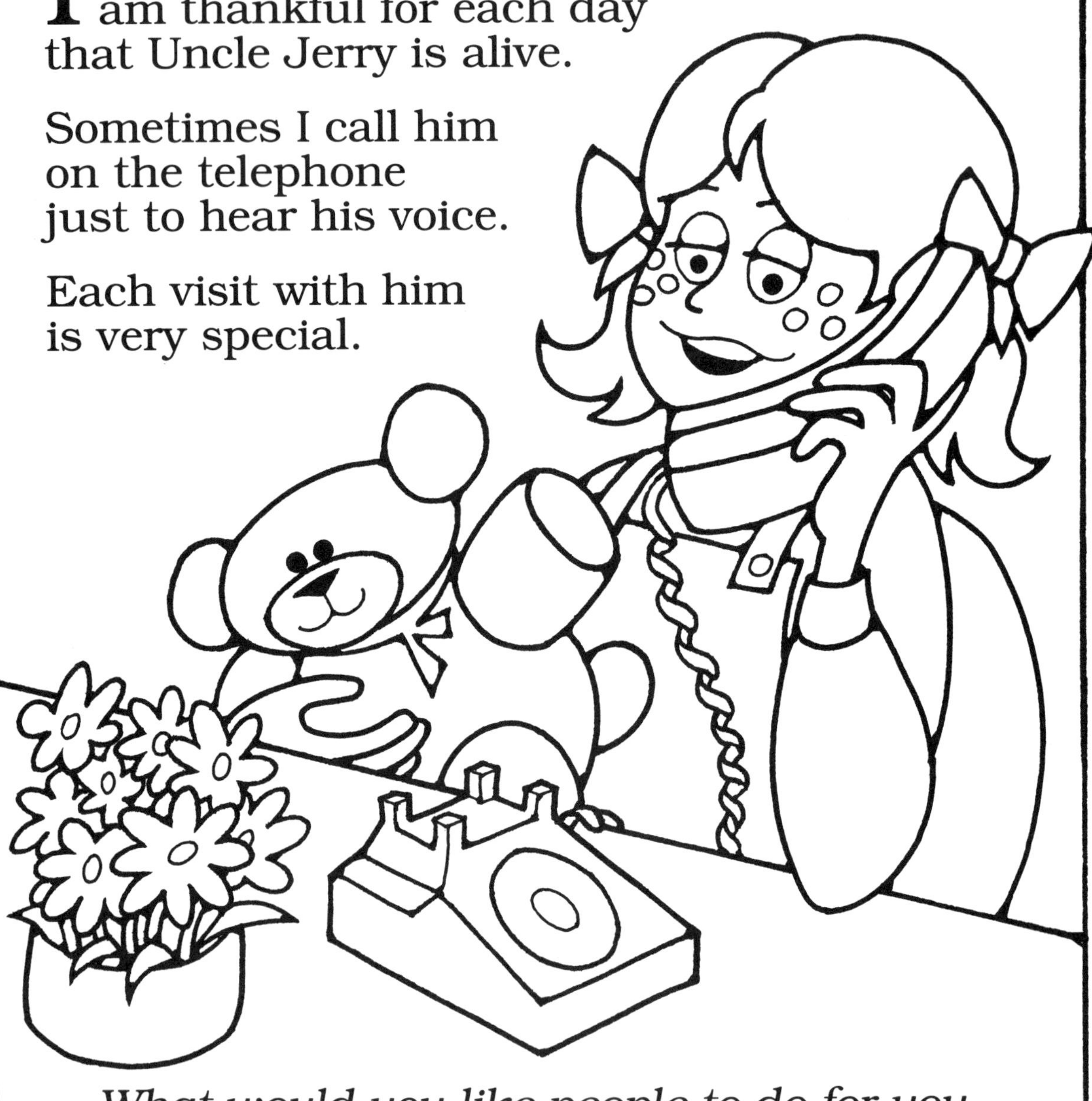

What would you like people to do for you if you were very sick? ______________________

____

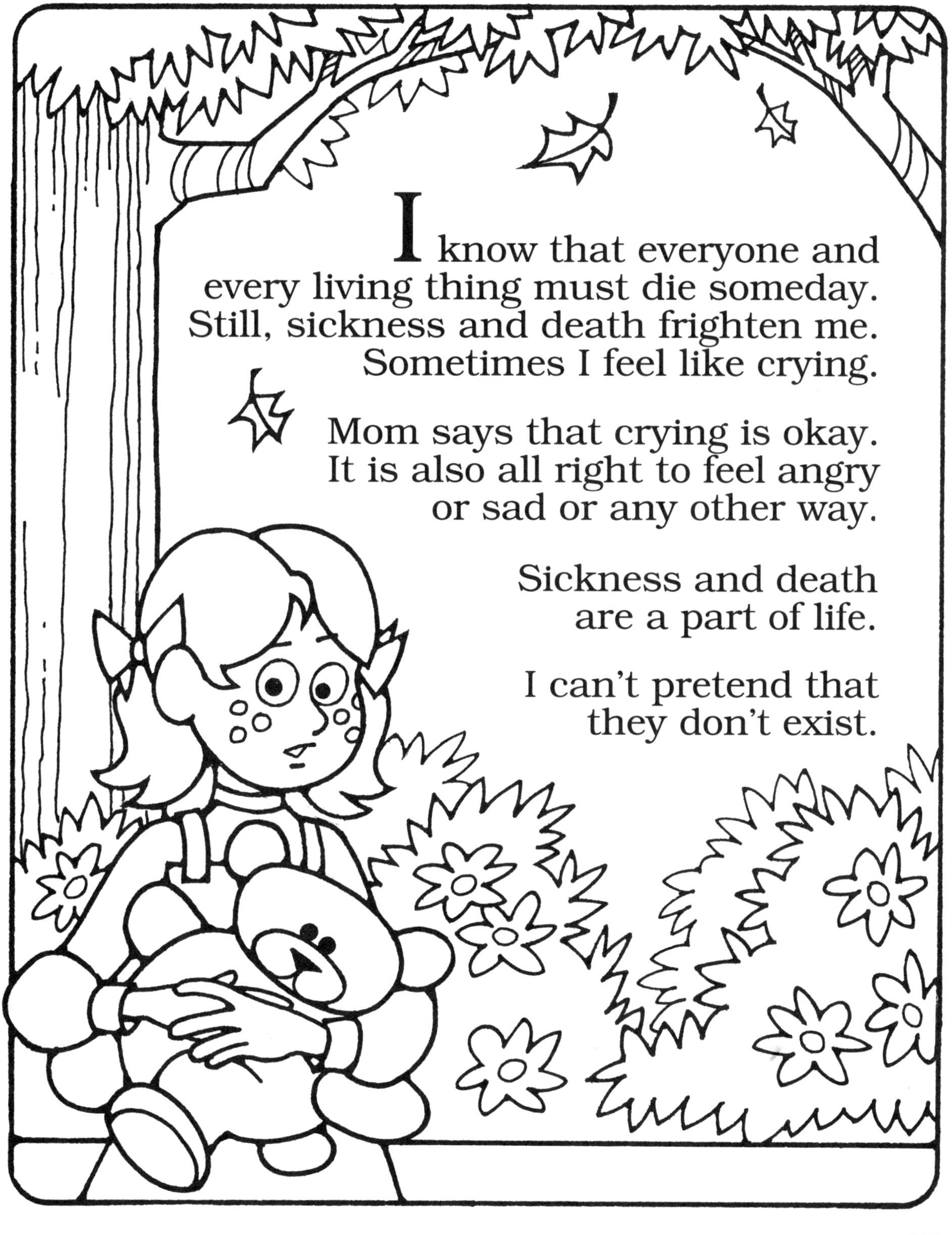

I know that everyone and every living thing must die someday. Still, sickness and death frighten me. Sometimes I feel like crying.

Mom says that crying is okay. It is also all right to feel angry or sad or any other way.

Sickness and death are a part of life.

I can't pretend that they don't exist.

My mom and I had a long talk about AIDS.

It felt good to tell her my feelings.

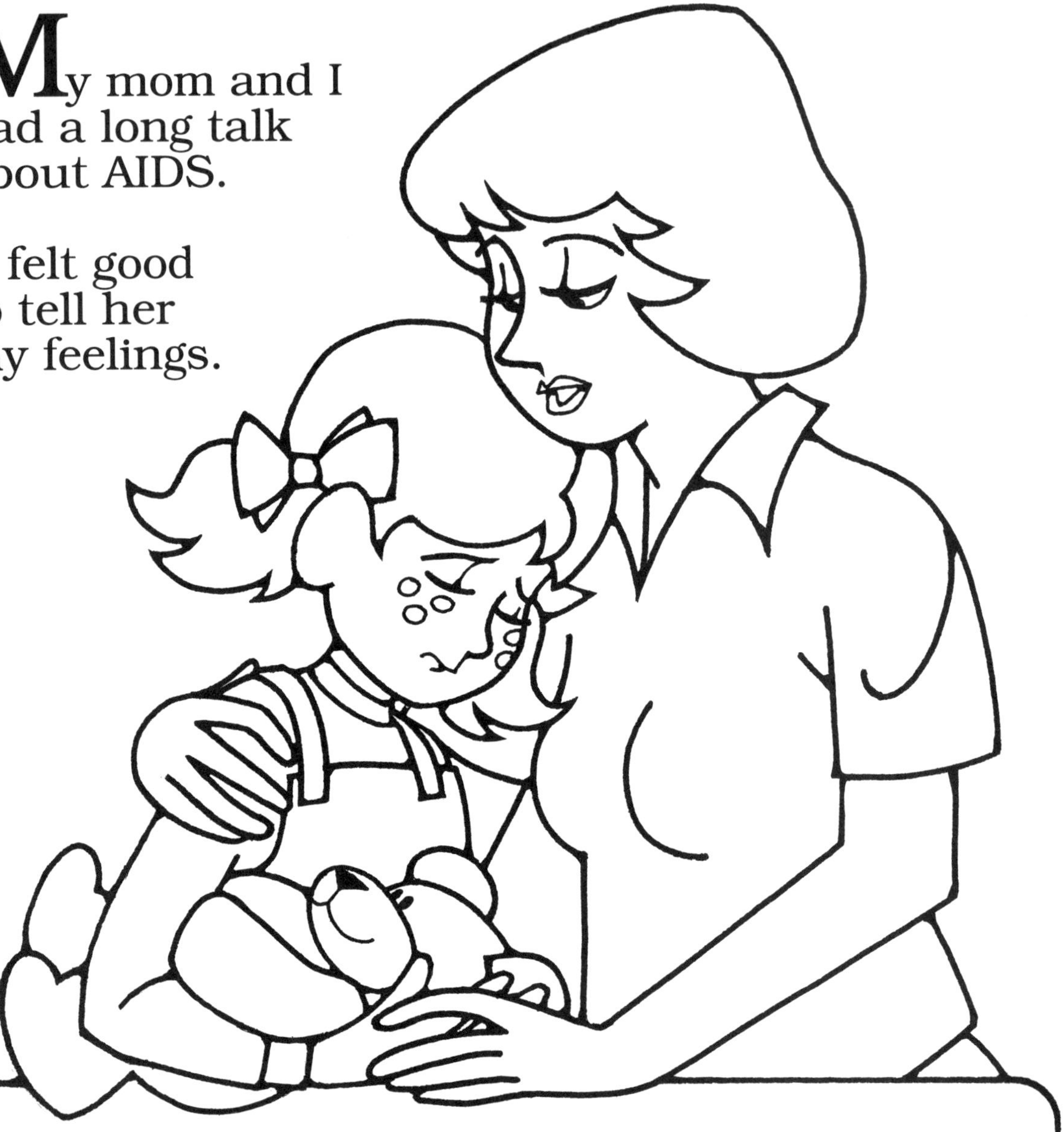

Who can you talk to about AIDS? ________

____

What questions would you like to ask?

____

It feels good to show my love
for Uncle Jerry.

I want him to know
that he is not alone.

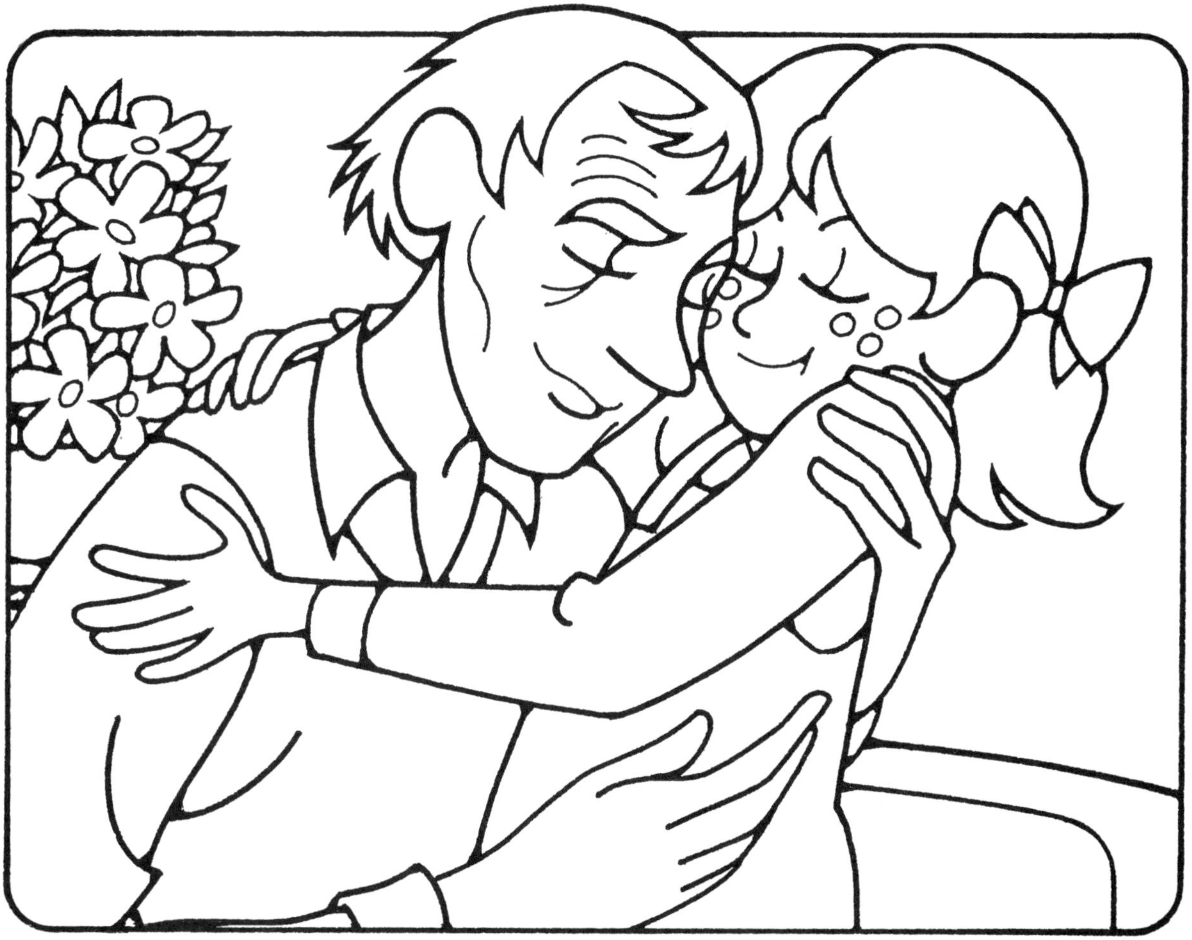

*How can you show someone with AIDS that you care?*____________________________

____

____

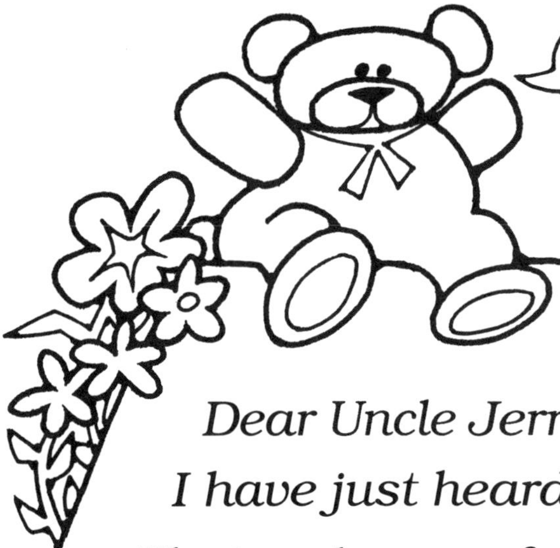

What would you like to say to Uncle Jerry?

Dear Uncle Jerry

I have just heard that you have AIDS.

That makes me feel very ____________________

I wonder if you feel ____________________

Does it ____________________

It would be nice if ____________________

I want you to know that ____________________

One question I have is ____________________

____

I wish ____________________

____

Your ____________________

____

Check the activities on the following list that put KT and her mother in danger of catching AIDS from Uncle Jerry.

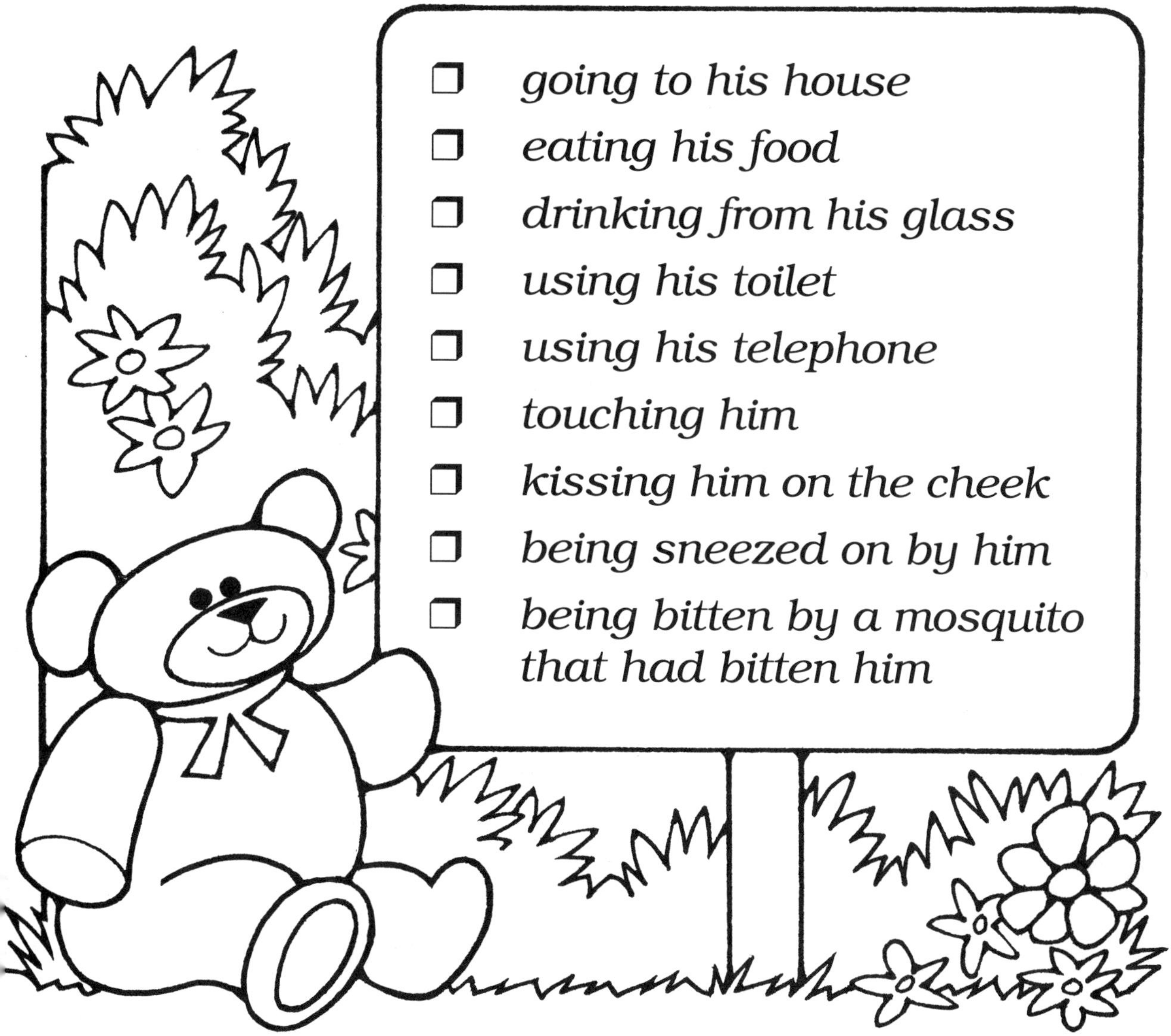

- ❒ *going to his house*
- ❒ *eating his food*
- ❒ *drinking from his glass*
- ❒ *using his toilet*
- ❒ *using his telephone*
- ❒ *touching him*
- ❒ *kissing him on the cheek*
- ❒ *being sneezed on by him*
- ❒ *being bitten by a mosquito that had bitten him*

Are you afraid that you or a loved one has AIDS?______If so, why do you feel that way?

____

Phone toll free 1-800-682-0029 for additional information or to place an order.
Full return privileges on all titles. 300,000 IN PRINT, USED BY 5,000 SCHOOLS.

SPECIAL PACKAGE OFFERS

Counselor's 7 Pack • Activity Books #1 to #7	$39.15
Divorce Support 4 Pack • Activity Books #2 to #5	$22.60
Library 32 Pack • 4 of Activity Books #1 to #8	$175.00
AIDS Classroom Kit • (Photocopy Permit)	$344.95

50 Activity Book #8 • 1 Teaching Guide • 1 Photocopy Master
1 Life Before Death Workbook

This kit was developed for group presentations where low cost consumable materials are important.
The purchase of this kit carries the right to reproduce the Uncle Jerry Has AIDS book.
The license to photocopy is specific to the purchaser of one location (i.e. one *school* — not *district*).

ACTIVITY BOOKS FOR CHILDREN IN DISTRESS

Grade Appropriate K-6

TITLE	QUANTITY	PRICE	TOTAL
1. **Saying Goodbye** (Bereavement)	______	$5.95	______
2. **Let's Talk** (Early Divorce)	______	$5.95	______
3. **My Story** (Divorce & Remarriage)	______	$5.95	______
4. **Alone Together** (Single Parent)	______	$5.95	______
5. **All Together** (Blended Family)	______	$5.95	______
6. **Feeling Good** (Self Esteem)	______	$5.95	______
7. **My Secret** (Parent Drug Abuse)	______	$5.95	______
8. **Uncle Jerry Has AIDS** (Emotion)	______	$5.95	______

SUPPORTIVE REFERENCES FOR ADULTS

Death & Dying 4 Pack #1, #9, #10 & #11	______	$38.95	______
9. **Life & Death** (300 Quotes)	______	$13.95	______
10. **Life Before Death Workbook**	______	$13.95	______
11. **Caregiver's Handbook**	______	$6.95	______

TOTAL CHARGES ______
Shipping Charge - Refer to Catalogue ______
G.S.T. 7% ______
TOTAL BILLING ______

FULL REMITTANCE MUST ACCOMPANY ORDERS FOR $30.00 OR LESS

SPECIAL INSTRUCTIONS: Purchase Order No., Shipping Instructions

Name ______ Phone ______ Fax ______
Organization ______
Street ______
City ______ Province ______ Postal Code ______

MARVIN MELNYK ASSOCIATES LTD.
P.O. Box 220, Queenston, ON L0S 1L0 • Phone: 1-416-262-4964 • Fax: 1-416-262-5303